"In this simple and elegantly crafted book, Chloe Isidora helps you to restore beauty and reverence to your daily life. Filled with rituals and ceremonies for different occasions and situations, and some divine recipes, it tenderly guides you into a more soulful, kinder relationship with yourself. A book to cherish indeed."

Alexandra Pope and Sjanie Hugo Wurlitzer, co-directors of Red School and co-authors of *Wild Power: Discover the Magic of Your Menstrual Cycle and Awaken the Feminine Path to Power.*

"Throughout history, rituals and ceremonies have always played a healing part in our lives, yet we have forgotten their importance. Chloe's gentle yet deep approach is the perfect way to re-introduce them into our lives. For health, emotional support and a sprinkle of magic, these beautiful offerings are suitable for anyone who values the nourishment of spirit."

Emma Cannon, fertility and women's health expert, acupuncturist and author.

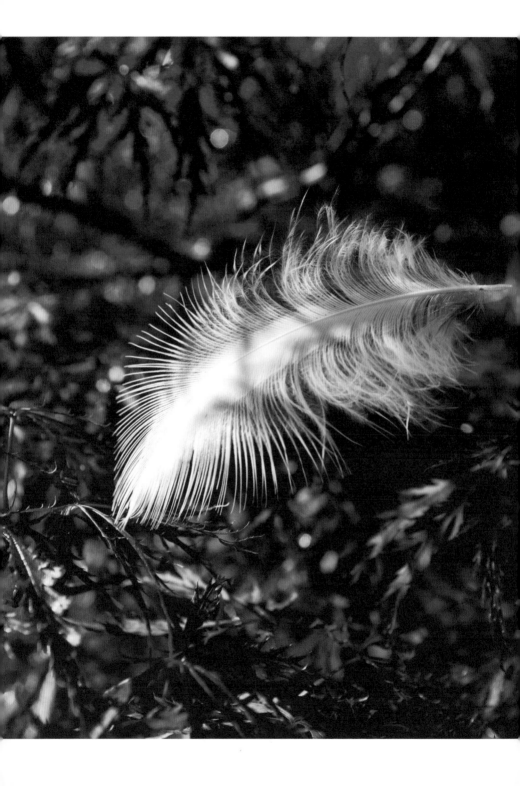

Sacred Self-care

Everyday rituals for a more
joyful and meaningful life

Chloe Isidora

Dedicated to the love affair of the heart

First published in Great Britain in 2019 by Aster, an imprint of Octopus Publishing Group Ltd
Carmelite House
50 Victoria Embankment
London EC4Y 0DZ
www.octopusbooks.co.uk
www.octopusbooksusa.com

An Hachette UK Company
www.hachette.co.uk

This edition published in 2023

Distributed in the US by
Hachette Book Group
1290 Avenue of the Americas
4th and 5th Floors
New York, NY 10104

Distributed in Canada by
Canadian Manda Group
664 Annette St.
Toronto, Ontario, Canada M6S 2C8

ISBN 978-1-78325-594-8

Printed and bound in China

10 9 8 7 6 5 4 3 2 1

All reasonable care has been taken in the preparation of this book, but the information it contains is not intended to take the place of any advice, counselling or treatment given by a qualified practitioner.

While all exercises and practices in this book are completely safe if followed correctly, you must consult a specialist before making any changes to your diet, lifestyle or health and fitness regime, and seek professional advice if you have any existing conditions or concerns.

Any application of the ideas and information contained in this book is at the reader's sole discretion and risk.

Consultant Publisher: Kate Adams
Editor: Ella Parsons
Copy Editor: Caroline Taggart
Art Director: Yasia Williams-Leedham
Photographer: Gustavo Papaleo
Production Manager: Lisa Pinnell

Geometry symbols: Sollex/Shutterstock

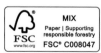

CONTENTS

Introduction

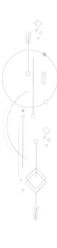

This is my story – the story of how I transitioned from the world of high fashion into the mystery of energy, healing, magic and transformation. In this book I have gathered together all the tools and practices I connect with, and many that I wish I'd been taught from an early age.

To set the scene, it all began when I was working as fashion editor for a highly creative magazine. At the time I wore only high heels, I had dyed jet-black hair and my staple wardrobe was Prada and Miu Miu. I was in a toxic relationship and I was completely addicted to the drama and pain that went along with it. In a nutshell, I was not happy.

One day an incredibly glamorous woman walked into the office – probably the chicest woman I have ever met. She was a friend of my boss and had come to borrow my Prada discount card. Off we went and started chatting, and it turned out to be one of those magical, serendipitous moments: we discovered we had the same birthday and out of nowhere I asked whether she knew of any healers. In that moment she put me in touch with my first Shaman.

A Shaman is a healer, an Earth keeper, a bridge between the natural and supernatural worlds. A person who reaches altered states of consciousness to interact with the invisible world and gain wisdom and insights. Believing that Spirit is alive in everything, a Shaman calls upon Nature energies, Earth energies and the elements, showing respect for Mother Earth and all sentient beings. Most of all, Shamans strive to create balance and harmony and walk the path of beauty.

The Shaman I was put in touch with was called Wendy, and she worked with me for many years. During that time she suggested I enrol on a course called the Hoffman Process, which assists in identifying negative behavioural patterns of feeling unloved and unlovable – patterns that have often been passed down from generation to generation. The aim is to come to forgiveness and acceptance for ourselves and others.

The course was seven days in a countryside house far away from modern life, with no mobile phones and no opportunity to back out! It was the first deep-healing retreat I had experienced: back then I had never done any kind of meditation or process work and so it was something of a shock. I was totally resistant – the only thing that kept me there was my implicit trust that Wendy knew what was good for me.

At the end of the week, by some miracle I'd managed to let go a little bit of my initial resistance. I began to soften and be receptive and I had an experience during a meditation that I will never forget. I felt my heart exploding and opening with light – it was extraordinary and exhilarating. The sensation was so new, my whole body was rushing and buzzing; I was on a natural high.

The next pivotal point was taking part in an Ayahuasca ceremony with my Shamanic healer. Ayahuasca is a vine that comes from the Amazon jungle, a powerful hallucinogenic that has been used since ancient times for the purpose of healing and transformation. During my first ceremony I had huge expectations of having visions: I thought the Ayahuasca would tell me how my life would unfold and what my path was. But literally nothing happened: no visions, no out-of-body experiences, nothing. I was furious. When the ceremony was complete, I left the ceremonial yurt and found myself back at the house where we were staying. There on the table was a copy of Ram Dass's book *Be Here Now*, and I opened it randomly to a page that said, "It didn't work, it didn't work on me." I thought, "Typical!" Even the book confirmed that my experience was a complete waste. And then something happened that changed the direction of my life instantly. Wendy said, "Chloe, maybe one day you will want to do what I'm doing."

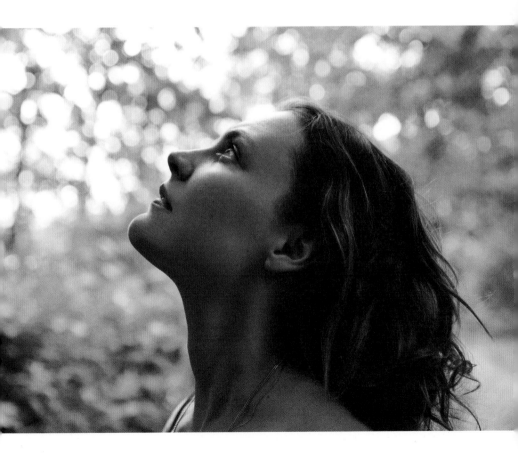

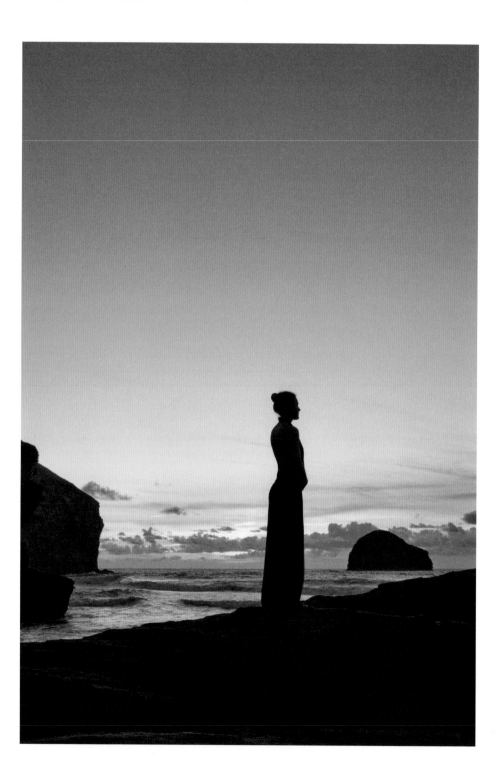

Back then I was so insecure I would never have said I had a calling or wish to be a healer and work with energy; I didn't even know what a calling was. I had no idea there were places you could go to learn about energy work, or that you could be initiated into a healing lineage. I thought you had to be born gifted with magical powers, and that there was no hope for me. But once Wendy made that suggestion, the door of possibility opened and I was beside myself with excitement. I shared with her that secretly this was exactly what I wanted to do. She probed further, asking what part of her sessions I liked best.

"The part where you rattle and use a pendulum," I replied.

"Ah, that's the Shamanic work," she said, smiling. "If you want to learn this, it's best to study with the Four Winds Society." And that's how I found myself enrolling in Shaman school.

But still, my life so far had been immersed in fashion. Even since I was a teenager, working in fashion was all I had ever wanted to do. I had been a fashion editor for ten years, working on shoots with incredible photographers. On paper I had my dream job, but in reality I was miserable. I had lost my passion and drive. I felt like a hamster caught in the spinning wheel, running over the same old ground, doing the same old thing and having the same conversations. I remember thinking, "There must be more to life than this."

And so in September 2013, I flew to New York City, got on a train to upstate New York and headed off to the Omega Institute, where the classes were to be based. The Four Winds Society is a renowned school of energy medicine. Its founder, Dr Alberto Villoldo, created the Light Body School, which is a combination of ancient Shamanic wisdom teachings, nutrition and neuroscience.

The first course I participated in was "The South", during which we were encouraged to connect to the energy of the serpent, imagining ourselves shedding our skin the same way a snake does. We were guided through many processes to identify our core wounds, fears and what was holding us back. Over the week I discovered that I felt completely worthless and that I was living with a sense of fear and lack. I was quite shocked to find out that these beliefs were running my life, and that every decision was coming from a place of fear – I'd had no idea.

Throughout the week I was desperate for a mystical experience. There were many advanced students in the class, and there was a lot of "Did you see her aura?", "Did you feel that?", "Did you see that energy?" going on. I was mad with jealousy as my answer was always "No" and my longing for a spiritual and mystical experience was heart-wrenching. I sobbed most of the week and had terrible headaches.

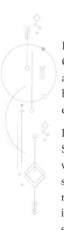

I'll always remember how supportive Alberto Villoldo was to me during that time. One day when I couldn't stop crying he took me by the arm, walked with me through a path lined with trees and said in his soothing voice, "Chloe, one day you will look back on this moment and realize it is now you who are taking another by the arm and encouraging them." He spoke kindly and gently, yet I didn't believe him.

In the class there was a beautiful woman named Aravel, who had long braided hair. She was always smiling and dancing; she was magnetic. I was drawn to her energy and wanted to be around her as much as possible. When she heard about my headaches she gave me two beautiful crystal skulls, telling me to hold on to them to see how they made me feel. I discovered she was a crystalline consciousness healer and so I booked in for a session with her. The session was held in a boiling hot tent, but as soon as she started the energy work my whole body became freezing cold. The experience was visceral. After the session I felt as if I had hypervision: the grass, blue sky, fluffy clouds, tiny birds and rabbits I saw looked crystal clear, clearer than I had ever seen them before. I knew something big had happened.

Crystalline consciousness, like all energy healing, is almost impossible to explain; you must experience it to understand it fully, but I will do my best! If we imagine ourselves as computers that are in need of a software update, essentially crystalline consciousness is the new software updating and upgrading our physical and angelic DNA. It assists in clearing out old stuff and aligning unconditional love with our true nature and opening up our Divine gifts.

On the last day of Light Body School, I vividly remember Alberto saying to the whole class, "Don't be surprised if your life changes when you go home." How right he was! In the space of a week my life unravelled.

I arrived home from New York on a Sunday evening. My boyfriend came over. For the past few months we had been going through a rocky patch, but I always thought we would survive it, as I truly believed he was "The One" and we would get married and have babies. That evening he said he couldn't continue and broke off our three-year relationship. I was devastated. The following day I went in to work to be told that a new fashion director was joining the magazine and I would be replaced by her chosen fashion editor. Within the space of not even a week, my identity was completely stripped. I was shattered into thousands of pieces, heartbroken and inconsolable, raging and confused. Losing my job I could just about handle, but losing the relationship was my worst nightmare coming true.

Out of the blue, Aravel called me from California. In floods of tears I told her what had happened. She said, "So, are you coming to San Francisco to the Shamanic Crystalline Consciousness course?" I had wanted to go from the moment she first mentioned it back in New York, but hadn't thought I would be able to get the time off work. That was no longer a problem. In the heat of the moment I said, "Yes, I'm coming!" But when she asked what I would do afterward, another flood of tears erupted. I had no idea. "Well, would you like to come and be my apprentice?" Really? That could be a possibility, I thought to myself.

Interestingly, that New Moon I had written down my wishes. I had wished, with gratitude, for a spiritual teacher: "Thank you for sending me a spiritual teacher." My wish had been granted!

So that's how my story begins. It's been a long journey to get to where I am now, with many more adventures. In the following pages I'll share some of the learnings, stories, tools, rituals and practices that have assisted my transformation.

My deepest wish is that what I share with you, and what you put into practice, will assist you in discovering your own inner truth and self-love in the face of the pressures you encounter in this modern world. I believe that learning to love and care for yourself is deeply healing and transformative work, and that when you consciously commit to this kind of self-care – and all the adventures that come with it – you will see how you might step fully into your own light.

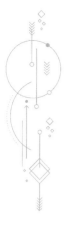

What Spirituality Means to Me

As you may have noticed already, from my story of how I came to the world of energy and healing, my sense of spirituality is not limited to my own upbringing or background. I was brought up in the Catholic religion, and Papa would take my sister and me to church every Sunday. I remember going to Sunday school, and I was confirmed, but I don't consider myself religious.

However, I do believe in a Divine presence that is bigger than my physical being and that resides within the deep well of my heart. Throughout this book I will use many names for what I experience this presence to be: God, Spirit, Source, Divine, Infinite Light, Great Spirit, Mother Father God, Goddess, the unnameable one, unconditional love. I believe there are multiple different paths we can follow to reach our own experience of the Divine: we just need to find the one that resonates with us the most.

I have travelled to many places in the world seeking understanding and ways of connecting to that Divine presence. Like many people today, I have a sense of spirituality that crosses continents, time and even dimensions, and I believe that there is so much wisdom to be gained from ancient and indigenous traditions.

And so a number of the rituals and ceremonies that I will share with you in this book have been taught to me by practitioners from varied traditions, including Shamanic teachings from the Four Winds Society, menstrual empowerment from the Red School, wisdom from Sri Amma Bhagavan at the O&O Academy and teachings from Mother Nature herself.

Over the course of the book I will also introduce you to my favourite Archangels and Divine Beings, who I find incredibly supportive as I navigate modern life. I believe that our ancestors and the Spirits of the land guide us and should be honoured, along with the Earth itself; the elements of water, fire, air and ether; and the winds that come from the four directions of the compass. All offer us connection, the potential for growth, understanding, wonder and transformation.

But most of all, for me, spirituality is a deep love affair of the heart. I would say that Nature is my temple and where I receive the deepest healing, and that I find my empowerment in the natural rhythm of my menstrual cycle. All of the practices in the book are about coming home to myself, about feeling and experiencing the Divine that lives within me. I encourage you to try all the rituals and ceremonies laid out in this book, and to discover which ones resonate most with you. My heartfelt wish is that you also are able to connect to the Divine that lives within you.

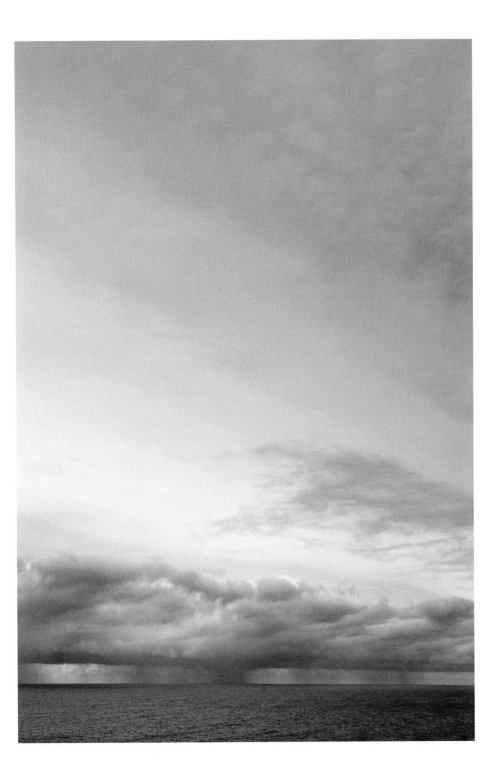

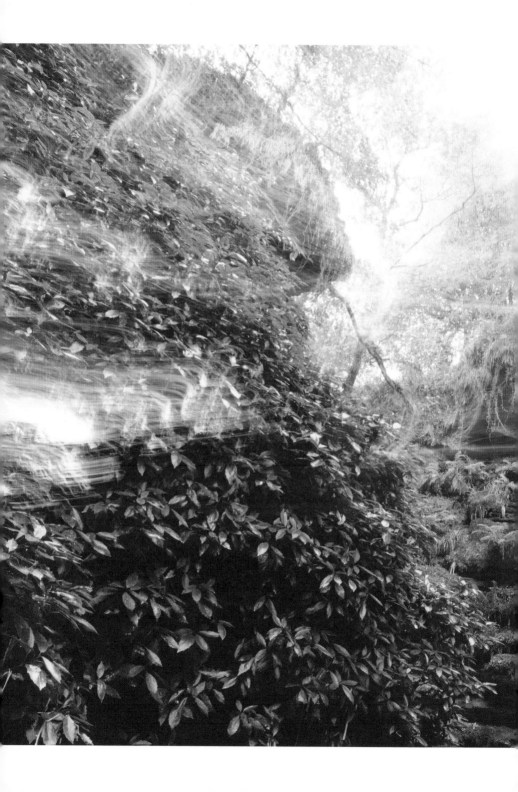

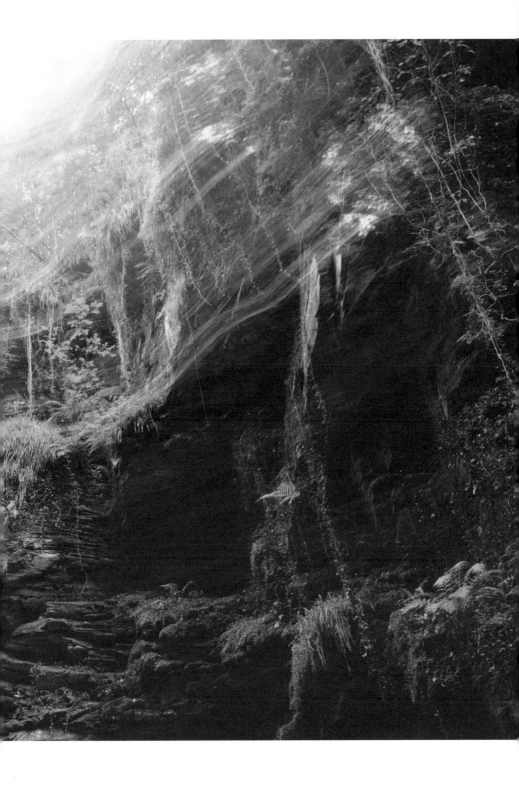

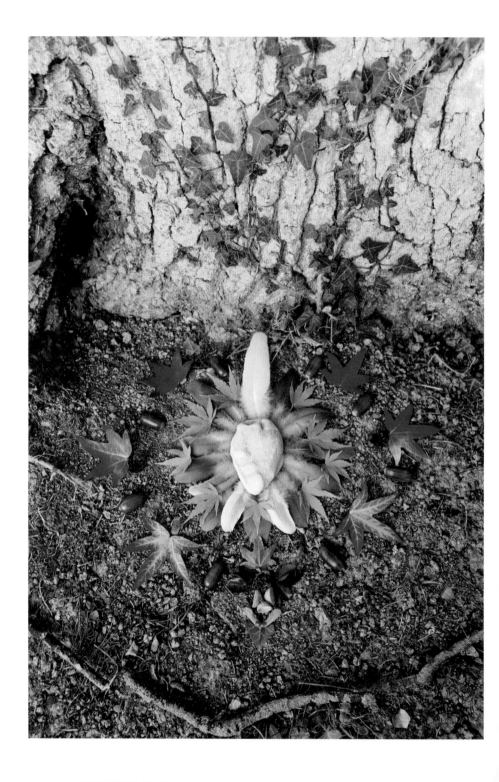

What Is Sacred Self-care?

For me, sacred self-care is about giving the most exquisite, impeccable love and care that you possibly can to yourself. It's about acknowledging your inner fears and shadows, allowing them space to surface so that you are no longer run by them. It's about bringing yourself from your mind into your body to feel what's there and to nurture yourself tenderly.

How can you create loving care in every situation? By creating space for pleasure and play. Weaving magic and miracles throughout your day. Choosing to be in your joy, choosing to love yourself and be in love with yourself, choosing to say yes to life. Being open, honest and truthful with yourself.

Throughout my day I engage in self-love and self-care practices, from being in the shower to washing my hands, eating food, sitting in meditation, dancing around – the list goes on and on. I have found ways that feel good to me. Becoming my own mother, lover and friend. Loving my body, honouring my mind, respecting all my emotions. All-singing, all-dancing, all-playing and sometimes all-crying!

When I was in my teens at boarding school I was forever writing depression lists – I never thought to write a list of the things I was grateful for. I was so busy focusing on what was wrong in my life that I didn't consider taking the time to focus on what was right. I was horribly mean to my body, bullying myself, thinking I was not pretty enough, not clever enough, not popular enough, not good enough.

One day, the penny dropped that I had a choice. I could choose to live a happy life or continue to live in my suffering. I'm not suggesting glazing over things that hurt – no, because there is gold there. There is a lesson every time a part of our Self is revealed to us. But we can choose to attach ourselves to suffering, or allow it to move through us.

Sacred self-care works on all levels:

• **Caring for your body** – finding the exercise and movement that you enjoy. I really don't like gym stuff, and didn't like yoga that much, either, until I found Kundalini yoga; now I start my day with a home Kundalini practice. I also love to dance and stretch.

• **Caring for your mind and emotions** – noticing and acknowledging thoughts when they appear throughout the day. Speaking out loud and asking yourself what's up. Just as you would with a friend, holding yourself through the emotional process and asking yourself what you need. Choosing not to give yourself such a hard time and letting yourself feel emotion, from ecstatic joy to raging anger!

• **Caring for your soul and spirit** – taking lots of time to be by yourself, to sit in silence and stillness. Being in Nature. Choosing to be grateful for all that you have and all that you no longer have. Offering your heart's work.

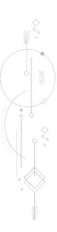

What Is a Ritual and What Is a Ceremony?

Woven together in this book are the many ceremonies and rituals that have become an integral part of my practice. When we create a ritual or a ceremony, we are consciously choosing to co-create with Spirit. You're allowing your human Self, with your own ideas and agendas, to step out of the way and are inviting and creating space for the Divine to guide you. When we work with Spirit in this way we are opening for magic to happen.

There is a difference between a ritual and a ceremony. A ritual implies repetition. Daily ritual could be having a cup of coffee at the same time in the same coffee shop or eating dinner at 7pm: something that is done at a similar time and has a fixed formula. We may not be aware of these habits, but they create structure to our day. If we choose to turn these habits into self-caring rituals and infuse them with meaning, purpose and connectivity, we can transform mundane moments into magic sacredness.

The self-loving rituals that prepare me for my day ahead include morning movement, meditation and an energetic shower cleansing. Throughout the day I wash my hands in golden liquid light, bless my food and drink and at night offer prayers and gratitude. Many rituals can be done alone, although some may be in the company of others.

A ceremony, on the other hand, is more like a rite of passage, marking a moment of change, growth or transformation. A birthday or a wedding is a rite of passage and a ceremony, usually involving other people. A ceremony is alive and interactive and often adapts to people and places; it evolves, flows and changes when it needs to.

I believe that when we offer a ceremony or a ritual we are weaving together a sacred container that invites us to connect to Source, to the Divine, to Spirit. When we call upon the invisible realms and engage in ceremony and ritual, we honour Spirit and remember we are connected to something bigger than ourselves. This is where magic and miracles can happen; a moment to remember that we are all part of all creation.

With any ceremony or ritual, I always start with great reverence, speaking an opening prayer, calling, welcoming and honouring Father and Mother God and Goddess, the Winds of the South, West, North and East, Mama Earth and all her relations, Father Sun, Grandmother Moon and my Spirit teams and lineages. I will share my personal prayer a little further on.

All the ceremonies and rituals in these pages are dedicated to sacred self-care. And while many of them can be done by both men and women, the book has been created with women in mind, to support the natural rhythms and cycles and to deepen into the feminine ways.

I believe that sacred self-care takes commitment, self-devotion and the willingness to say yes to yourself. No one else can do this for you. It's about choosing yourself, choosing to honour yourself, choosing to respect and love yourself. Are you ready to choose *you*? Take a moment to repeat the following:

I am ready to commit to myself.

I am ready to set aside time for myself.

I am ready to love myself.

I am ready to respect myself.

I am ready to honour myself.

I am ready to treat myself as sacred.

I am ready to say YES to being ME.

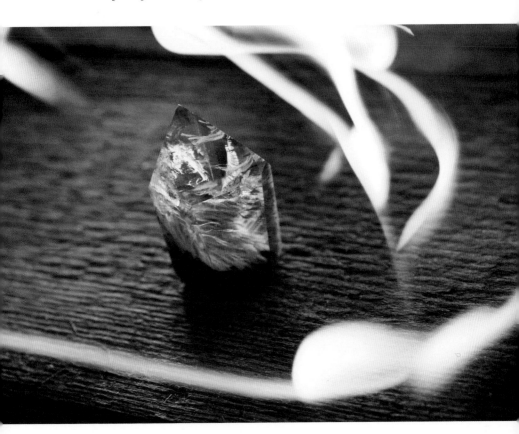

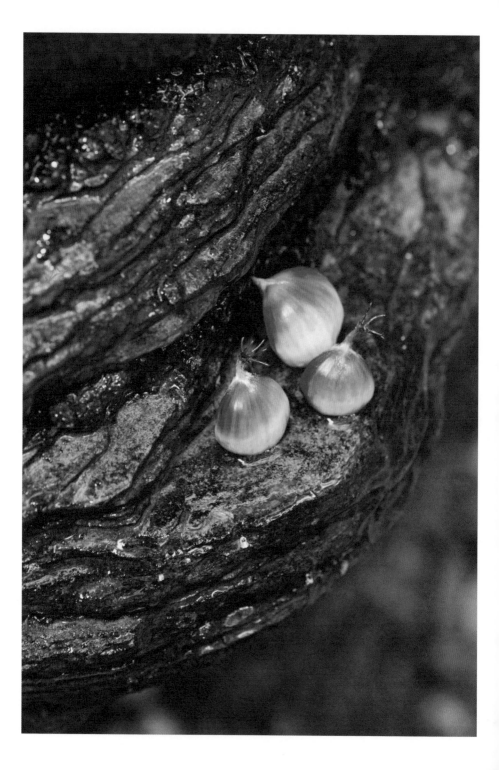

Setting Your Intention

Before starting any practice, I first set an intention. An intention is the essence of your wish, prayer or desire. Setting an intention gives focused, decisive energy to that wish, which is then amplified by the practice. I love the saying "Energy goes where your attention flows", meaning that the more we focus our attention on something, the bigger it will become. Intentions are made consciously and are then released, so that you are not attached to a specific outcome but trust that the highest good will come from your intention.

For example, before I started writing I set the intention that this book would uplift, inspire, empower and bring heart connection to its readers. You can set an intention for anything: in the morning you might set the intention for a day filled with joy and creativity; before a meeting you might set the intention that it will be filled with clarity.

◎ Take a moment and close your eyes. Place your left hand on your heart, if you choose, and ask yourself:

"What is my intention? What is my wish?"

Tuning In

I will use this phrase throughout the book, at the beginning of every meditation and practice. What I mean by "tuning in" is coming into presence and awareness of yourself and where you are, and coming into inner stillness to feel your Divine essence. I suggest that you read this practice through and then go ahead and try it.

◎ Sit on the floor or on a chair, in an upright position with your spine straight. Close your eyes and place your left hand on your heart or have your hands on your lap.

◎ Relax your shoulders, allow your arms to become heavy, invite your belly to soften and puff out. Feel your weight in your sitting bones, feel yourself connected to the floor or chair.

◎ Take three long, slow, deep breaths, breathing in for a count of four and out for a count of four. Soften your body again.

◎ Gently bring your attention to rest on your heart centre and simply notice what you feel there – what sensations or feelings are you aware of? This is coming into presence with yourself.

◎ Rest your attention here in your heart for a few minutes or for as long as you like. Simply notice the sensations in your body. Notice how you feel.

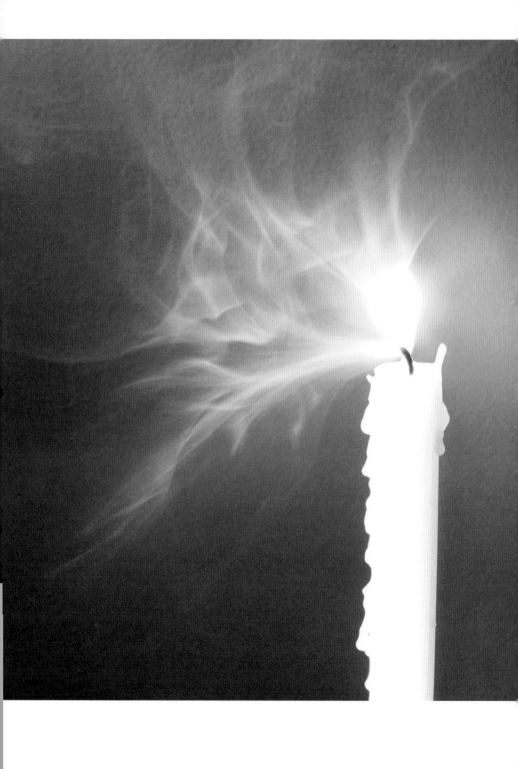

Chapter I

Creating Sacred Space

In this chapter we will be looking at how to create sacred space in your environment by physically and energetically preparing it. It is important to cleanse and clear your environment, both as a simple act of self-care and to give you a space where you can sit quietly, let the busy energy of the day drop away and connect with yourself.

It is very nourishing to create sacred spaces in our homes; they help us to be receptive to the subtle energies around us and give us room to be with our inner thoughts and emotions. Having a place for our favourite crystals, for example, encourages us to bring our attention to their beauty and to connect with their energy, while lighting a candle at the end of the day becomes a moment for transitioning into a more restful energy. We can also cleanse our own energy with simple rituals, breathing exercises and movement.

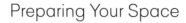

Preparing Your Space

Before engaging in any sacred work, it is important to set the scene both physically and energetically. I call it "tuning in" (see page 21). We attune ourselves to the subtle, and invisible, energies that are all around us. Our bodies are like tuning forks; we are constantly receiving information and sensing different energies, but how often do we tune in?

One way to begin attuning yourself to energy is to notice how you feel when you walk into certain spaces or rooms. Do you feel comfortable? Relaxed? On edge? Start noticing how you feel everywhere you go. What is your body telling you?

At home I run quite a tight energetic container: often when people come in they say they feel very relaxed, as if they had just stepped into an oasis from the outside world. My friend Jayne calls it "the heart home". My home feels like this to people who come over because I'm continually attuning the energy in my home.

Ingredients

natural cleaning products, fresh flowers, music, white sage (see page 186), bowl, matches, palo santo (see page 186), blessing spray (see page 27) or incense (optional)

◎ Physically clean and clear your space. Imagine you have guests visiting and you want the house to be super-tidy. Put away anything that doesn't need to be out, vacuum the floor, plump up the cushions, add fresh flowers. Having too many things around can create stagnant energy, so we want to move it and allow the energy to circulate freely.

◎ Now it's time to clear the space energetically. First, open a window to allow the old energy to leave. Play some music: the sound of sacred songs attunes the vibrations that ripple through the atmosphere so that the air hums with sacred sounds. I play the chant *Om Namah Shivaya* to build energy and create a sacred environment (see page 163).

◎ Now bring your focus to the sage, a powerful plant that assists in clearing denser energies. Thank her for cleansing and purifying your space. With a bowl underneath to catch the falling ash, set the sage alight and then blow out the flame – the sage will smoke. Walk around the house while holding your intention to cleanse, clear and purify. Once you feel complete, press the sage into the bowl to stop the burning.

◎ Now light a stick of palo santo and wave this all around your space. As you are walking around, set your intention. Palo santo calls in sweetness and joy, so your intention could be to fill your home with joy, peace, beauty and love. You could also use a favourite incense or a homemade room blessing spray.

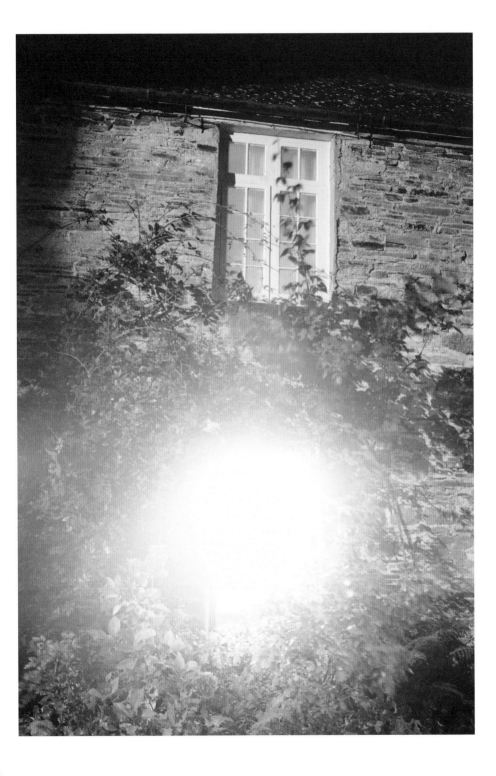

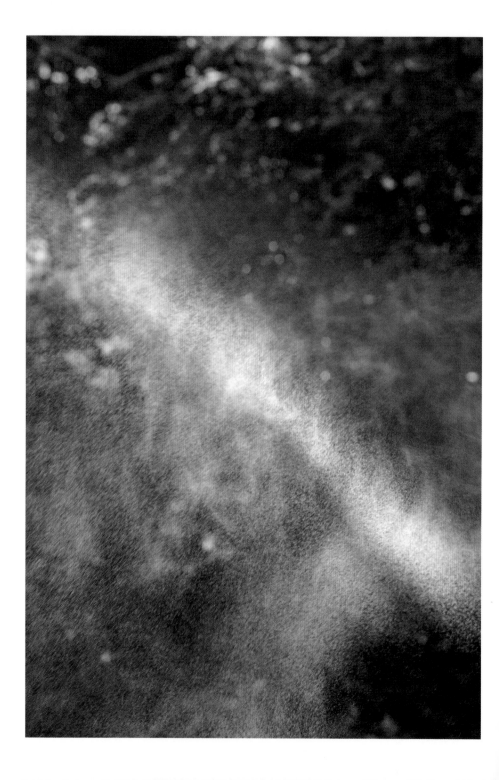

Blessing Your Home

Our homes give us shelter, keep us warm and look after us. But how often do we thank them? I like to imagine that my house is a living being (she's called Casa K): I thank her for looking after me and all who visit. I bless my home intentionally, calling in Earth energy, calling in the support and grace of the angelic realms and the highest vibration of love. Blessing your home can be done daily or when you feel it is necessary.

◎ Close your eyes and place your left hand on your heart. Send your breath in and out of your heart. Begin saying thank you. You could repeat the following, or adapt the wording as you wish:

"Thank you, beautiful home, for sheltering me, for keeping me safe. Thank you, Mama Earth, for supporting the foundations, thank you for your Earth energy infusing my home with radiance. Thank you, angels, for surrounding my home in a golden orb of light. Thank you for holding my home in the vibration of unconditional love. Blessed be and so it is."

Room Blessing Spray

You can also use a water-based essential oil spray to cleanse and clear your space. I tend to make this spray on a New or Full Moon for extra potency (see page 120).

Ingredients

glass bottle with spray lid, a mixture of the following essential oils: rosemary, frankincense, lavender and clary sage, blessed water (see page 41)

◎ Tune in. Set your intention for the spray by saying something like:

"I intend to make a blessing spray that cleanses, purifies and brings in the highest frequency of unconditional love."

◎ Add the oils to the bottle first. Use your intuition as to how many drops you need – smell as you go along. I can tell when the mix is complete, as my heart softens and opens. Do you have a sense that it is complete?

◎ When you are ready, add the blessed water. Pop the spray lid on. Close your eyes and give your room a spritz. How do you feel?

You could also create a spray to invoke love, creativity, joy. Just use these essential oils:
to invoke love – rose otto, frankincense, jasmine, ginger, neroli
to invoke creativity – clary sage, peppermint, mandarin, rosemary
to invoke celebration – rose geranium, frankincense, bergamot, lavender, neroli

When the Energy Feels Wonky!

Sometimes you might enter an environment that feels a bit "off". You might be uncomfortable or even scared and jumpy. Maybe you're staying somewhere new – in an unfamiliar hotel, perhaps – and something just doesn't feel right.

A friend once messaged me to say she was frightened in her house, she couldn't relax and was having trouble sleeping; she felt as if there was a negative energy and didn't feel safe. I shared this prayer with her, calling in the support of Archangel Michael. After the invocation my friend said that she felt a hundred times better.

Archangel Michael is considered the archangel of protection and courage. He represents the all-encompassing power and strength of the Divine and is often depicted with a shield and sword. Personally, I call upon Archangel Michael for protection, courage and strength – any time I feel the need. I always call upon him when I'm driving, for extra safety.

◎ Place your left hand on your heart and bring your attention and focus to your heart centre. Send your breath in and out of your heart. Call on the angelic realms, especially Archangel Michael; ask for his protection, his strength, grace and presence. Thank him for surrounding the space in a golden orb of light, so that it is held in the highest frequency of love and Divine light.

Preparing Your Body to Receive Spirit

Before a session, workshop, ceremony or ritual for myself or others, I always prepare my physical vessel and the space around me. By "vessel" I mean your body, your mind, your intentions and prayers. By doing this you are preparing all parts of yourself.

I have adapted this practice from different Kundalini yoga stretches and so, ideally, you need a yoga mat.

- Get into your body: loosen your muscles, lubricate your spine and iron out all the crinkly bits.

- Start by taking three long, slow and deep breaths, inhaling for a count of seven, and then exhaling for a count of seven.

- Sitting cross-legged, hold your ankles and move your spine forward and back, keeping your head parallel to the floor. Do this rocking motion for three minutes.

- Then move your hands to your knees and continue with the same movement, rocking back and forward and feeling a stretch in the middle of your back. Do this for another three minutes.

- Hold your arms up in a cactus shape, elbows level with the shoulders. Turn to the left and then to the right, breathing in as you turn to the left and out as you turn right. Keep this going for another three minutes.

- Take a moment to rest, placing your hands on your knees, and feel the new energy you have created.

- Roll your hips to the left and then to the right for another three minutes (if you're used to yoga, you'll recognize this as a Sufi Grind).

- Turn over on to your hands and knees and do a Cat-Cow stretch, first raising your face toward the ceiling and pushing your belly down toward the floor, breathing in. Then breathe out as you lower your head and arch your back up. Continue for another three minutes.

- Come to an upright kneeling position. Roll your shoulders forward and back, then bring your shoulders up to your ears and drop them down.

- Gently roll your neck three times to the left and three times to the right.

- Feel in your body where else you want to stretch, and then stretch freestyle.

- Consciously take three long, slow, deep breaths.

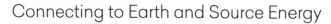

Connecting to Earth and Source Energy

This meditation is a great way of attuning to the energy of the Earth and Source. It is incredibly supportive and nourishes every part of your being. It is wonderful for cleansing or letting go of energy you no longer need, or for when you feel wobbly in yourself.

◎ Sit in a comfy, upright position with your back straight (it is important that you are comfortable, so if your back bothers you, lie down).

◎ Begin with three long, slow breaths. Let your shoulders become heavy, allow your arms to drop and feel your sitting bones on the floor or chair. Choose to relax your body and to let go.

◎ Bring your attention to your heart, and then drop your focus to the base of your spine. Set your intention to ground yourself and connect to the core of the Earth.

◎ Imagine that you are sitting outside in a beautiful, sacred space in Nature. Imagine there is a root unfurling from the base of your spine or roots growing down from your feet.

◎ Invite your root(s) to grow down and down through the soil, down through the bedrock, through the layers of minerals. Imagine the colours changing from yellow to orange to red as you keep going down, asking to be connected to the core of the Earth. Once there, imagine wrapping your root(s) around Earth's core three times.

◎ Ask Mama Earth to drain any energy from you that is not for your highest good. Soften your body and choose to let go. Feel a draining sensation as any dense energy is taken from you.

◎ Now, call in Earth's golden liquid light. Imagine this energy spiralling up from the centre of the Earth all the way up your root(s) and entering the base of your spine or the soles of your feet. Allow your whole body to be filled with golden liquid light.

◎ Now that you are grounded to the Earth, the next stage is to connect to Source. Imagine a thread of light spiralling up from the crown of your head toward the Cosmos. Set your intention to be connected to your own personal star and invite Source energy to shower down all around you. Imagine a white light enter the crown of your head and travel all the way down into the base of your spine.

◎ Close by thanking the Earth, Source and yourself, then take some deep breaths, wriggle your fingers and toes and, when you feel ready, blink your eyes open. Now you are connected to Heaven and Earth.

Creating an Altar

One of my favourite things to do is to create an altar. This is a place where you can set your intentions, pray, offer your dreams and wishes. It is a sacred space in your home that is an anchor point. You might create an altar for your Divine, your God or Goddess, or you might call in abundance, health and wellness. I love to include special items such as crystals, candles and things that I find in Nature, maybe feathers, rocks, sticks, leaves and pine cones.

Ingredients

an altar cloth or a beautiful piece of fabric, any items that you feel are sacred to you (such as crystals, rocks, fresh flowers, feathers, candles)

◎ Before you begin, take a few moments to tune in. What is your intention in creating this altar?

◎ Lay the altar cloth or fabric in your chosen space and begin placing the items on it. Think about what each item represents to you. Place all your pieces on the altar, creating something beautiful and aesthetically pleasing to you. Bring all your love, all your focus.

◎ Visit your altar every day. You may like to write down your prayers or wishes and place them under one of your objects. Keep checking with your altar: it is an extension of you – does anything need to be moved, taken away or added? Bring freshness and newness to your altar by offering fresh flowers.

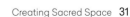

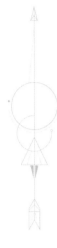

Opening Sacred Space

Now that we have created sacred space, and before we engage in any kind of sacred ceremony, ritual or healing, it is imperative to open it. By opening sacred space we are setting a strong, energetic container for only the highest energy of unconditional love to enter. We are calling on the elements, Mother Earth and Spirit.

Ingredients

candle, matches

◎ Light a candle and tune in.

◎ Say an opening prayer. You can use the following wording, or create your own version. Set your intention to speak from the heart.

"With great love, great honour and great respect I ask to open sacred space. I call upon you, Mama Earth, and thank you for the support, abundant nourishment and love you freely give me every day, I thank you for bringing all your relations, the stone people, the crystal people, the plant people, the two-legged, the four-legged, the winged, the creepy-crawlies, the elementals and the devas.

Calling upon the element of water, I thank you for your purification, for your ease and flow, for showing us the path of least resistance.

Calling upon the element of fire, thank you for your alchemy of transmutation and transformation, for the power and passion you bring.

Calling upon the element of air, you who are the sustainer of all life of every breath, thank you for your movement and continual presence.

Calling upon the element of ether, you who connect us to everything and everyone, you who weave all life together.

Calling upon Spirit, you who are known by a thousand names and who are unnameable. Mother, Father, God, Goddess and our star brothers and sisters. Calling upon my teams, my lineages, the angels and archangels. Thank you for opening and holding this space in the highest vibration of unconditional love for healing and transformation."

Closing Sacred Space

Once you have completed your sacred work, it is important to close sacred space. Thank all the elements for their support, for the healing they have offered, thank all the light beings. Speak from your heart and with gratitude.

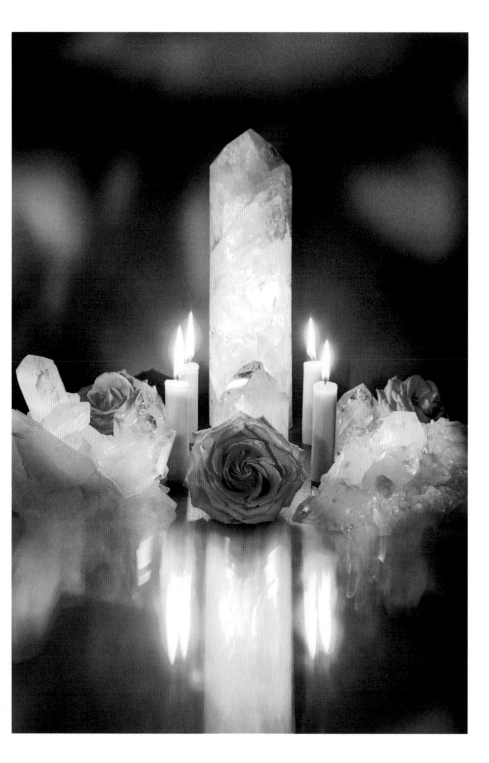

Chapter 2
Mundane Life into Magic Moments

In this chapter we explore how to weave a sense of magic and wonder into what might seem like mundane everyday tasks such as showering, washing our hands, making tea, cooking, eating and drinking.

What I find exciting about these practices is that we go about our normal life, but we look through a different lense: what might have seemed like a chore before is now filled with awe, all thanks to our intention and redirected focus. Absolutely everything we do can be infused with energy, with creativity, with love and devotion. Bringing awareness and presence into all that we do on a moment-to-moment basis creates a powerful shift and opens us to the magic and miracles of daily life.

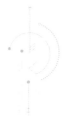

Waking Up to a Wonderful World

When we first open our eyes and stir in bed in the morning, we have an opportunity to consider how we want the day ahead to unfold. To choose what side of bed to get out of! The way to do this is to start the day in gratitude.

◎ Allow and invite everything and anything – no matter how big or small – to come up to the surface. Then speak your gratitude aloud.

"I'm so grateful for my super-comfy bed, I'm grateful for my soft sheets and my fluffy pillows, I'm grateful that the Sun is shining, I'm grateful that I woke up today!"

◎ Keep going for a minute or two or even longer. See what you notice. How do you feel?

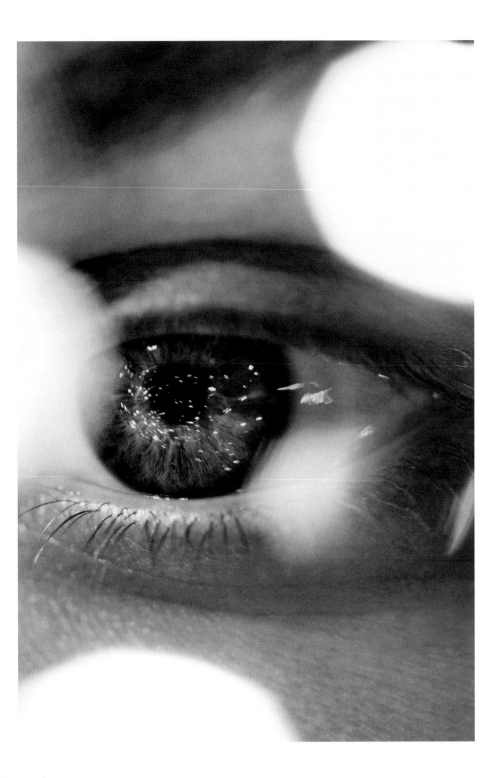

Stretching

This is a delicious way to start your day. It means taking time to listen to your body and moving and stretching in ways that feel good to you – not following anyone else's guidance, just listening to what your body wants. Freestyling to create movement and flexibility.

◎ Take a few minutes to stretch out your whole body, in any way that feels good to you. Stretch out your hips and shoulders, loosen your spine.

Morning Tea Ritual

The simple act of creating a tea ritual can set an uplifting tone for your day. When making your tea, view it as a moment you are gifting yourself, a moment of presence, relaxation and nourishment, a way of creating balance.

◎ Turn on the kettle. As the water is boiling, breathe in and out deeply, taking long, slow breaths.

◎ When the water is boiled, bring your full attention to it as you pour it into the cup or pot. Notice the steam rising, the tea leaves opening or the tea bag dancing in the water. Notice the tea changing the colour of the water and notice how you feel – all emotions are welcome.

◎ Before you take a sip, check in with your body to see whether you are relaxed or tense, then choose to relax any part of yourself that needs it.

◎ Now bring the cup up to your heart; take a moment to be grateful for the water – this water that gives you life and sustains you. Acknowledge the tea, which came from the Earth and took a whole host of people to get it to you, from producers to sellers.

◎ Close your eyes when you take the first sip. Be completely in the experience of drinking. Feel the warmth of the tea flowing down into your heart space. Notice what you feel.

◎ End with gratitude.

Showering in Golden Light

Energy hygiene is a big one for me. We often spend our days in busy environments, picking up on other people's energy, thoughts and feelings. This can often shape how we feel and, in the worst-case scenario, create heaviness. This energy is invisible to the eye, but can still have a profound effect on our day-to-day wellbeing. It can also be dealt with very quickly.

This shower ritual is something I do every morning or evening without even having to think about it. The purpose is to cleanse and clear your energy body from any dense, heavy energies you have picked up and to fill you with rejuvenating, restorative light.

◎ Begin by getting into the shower and turning on the water. Close your eyes, invite your body to soften and take three long, deep breaths. Consciously choose to connect to the energy of the water. Notice how your body reacts.

◎ In your own way, give thanks to the water, acknowledging that she is sacred, always taking the path of least resistance, that she washes, cleanses and purifies, that "water is life".

◎ Offer an internal prayer along the lines of:

"Dear Sacred Waters, thank you for cleansing, clearing and purifying me from any energies that are not aligned to my highest good, so I may start my day fresh and clear."

◎ Experience any heaviness falling away from your body and being washed down the plughole.

◎ Once you feel a sense of emptiness and letting go, visualize golden liquid light washing your whole body and filling up every cell of your being. Offer a prayer:

"Thank you for filling me with golden liquid light."

◎ Repeat front and back.

◎ As you leave the shower, imagine a golden orb of light surrounding you.

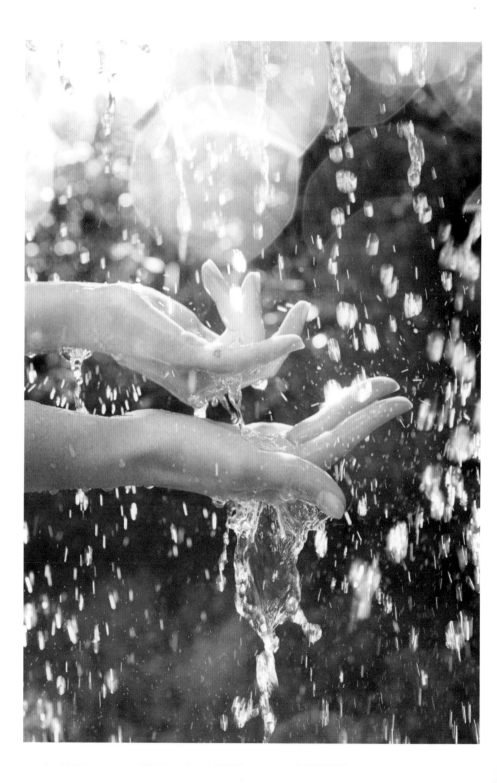

Washing Your Hands in Golden Liquid Light

Every time we wash our hands, we have the opportunity to cleanse, clear and bring freshness and vitality into our being. When I wash my hands, I imagine that golden liquid light is being poured over them at the same time as the water is flowing over. It keeps my hands energetically clear and clean as I go about my day.

◎ Turn on the tap and wash your hands as usual, then imagine that golden liquid light is pouring over them. Say, internally:

"Thank you for washing my hands in golden liquid light."

Water Blessing

Water is a sacred, living energy that carries the great flow of life; it is our most vital life-giving element and is to be honoured and respected. Water has a life-force energy that responds to the vibrations created when we talk out loud. So, when we bless the water, we are talking to the life-force energy, reminding the water of its own pure, clean, clear frequency, so that it becomes activated for healing and transformation.

◎ Placing your hand over a glass of water, give thanks to the water, honouring her as the sustainer of life and acknowledging that all water is sacred.

◎ Blow your gratitude into the water, blow your respect into the water, blow your love into the water.

◎ Drink, noticing how you feel when you drink blessed water.

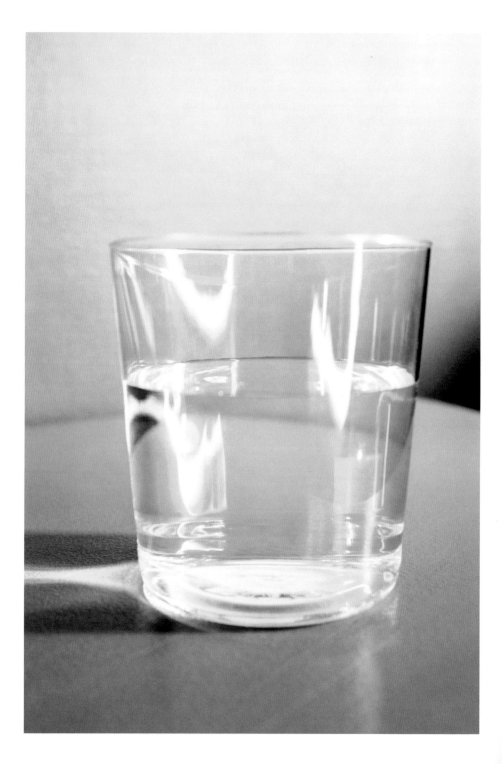

Food Blessing

This is a beautiful practice. It encourages us to feel gratitude every time we eat, reminding us that our food has come from the Earth and making us aware of all the various pathways it has taken to reach our plate. If we are eating vegetables, for example, we can think of the Earth that grew them, nourishing them with her soil, and of the water and Sun that fed and supported the vegetables to grow. Once they were ready, the vegetables were harvested, then packed up, sold, displayed in a shop, bought with money that needed to be earned and finally chopped and cooked! A whole chain of events had to happen to bring your food to your plate.

◎ Before you eat or drink, place your hands over the plate or bowl and bring all your awareness to the food in front of you.

◎ Close your eyes and internally say a prayer:

"Dear Source, infinite light, thank you for blessing this food. Dear Mama Earth, thank you for your nourishment and energy; thank you for this food that you have grown; thank you, Sun, water and soil. Thank you to the farmers who planted and harvested these vegetables; thank you to all the people involved in bringing this food to me; thank you to the shops that sold the food; thank you to the money that allowed me to buy this food; thank you to the people who have cooked and prepared this meal. Thank you for filling this food with love, which will only do me good."

Short version:

◎ *"This food that is filled with love and will only do me good, thank you, thank you, thank you."*

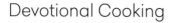

Devotional Cooking

I offered Seva, which means selfless service, at a Yoga Ashram. My job was to prepare the food for the chef to cook. Everything was done with great love and care. We would listen to mantras chanting in the background, prepping in silence and with focus.

While chopping, we would internally repeat the mantra *Om Namah Shivaya* (see page 163), which means "I bow to Shiva". By chanting this mantra we would connect to our inner Self, Divine love, grace and truth. This simple act expanded the vibration of the food, infusing it with love and devotion. I remember at one point I lost my focus and the chef looked at me and said in a sweet voice, "Cut this with love and devotion."

It's a beautiful way to be present while you are preparing any meal. You don't need to repeat the same mantra, you could make up your own. For example, "I infuse this food with love." By doing this, you make sure that all actions are coming from the heart with love and devotion, with pleasure and gratitude. Feeling that it is an honour to make the food.

People will notice without you saying a word. Intention is everything.

◎ Start by respecting your kitchen, by beginning with clean work surfaces and a clean and clear space.

◎ Set your intention that you are going to cook this food with love and devotion and that all who eat it will be blessed.

◎ With every chop of the knife, infuse the food with an enriching energy. Infuse it with joy, beauty, nourishment, inspiration, great health, happiness, generosity or integrity.

◎ Play devotional music if you like, or stay in silence. Avoid chit-chat with people. Try this as a focused meditation, thinking and feeling love as you prep and cook your meal.

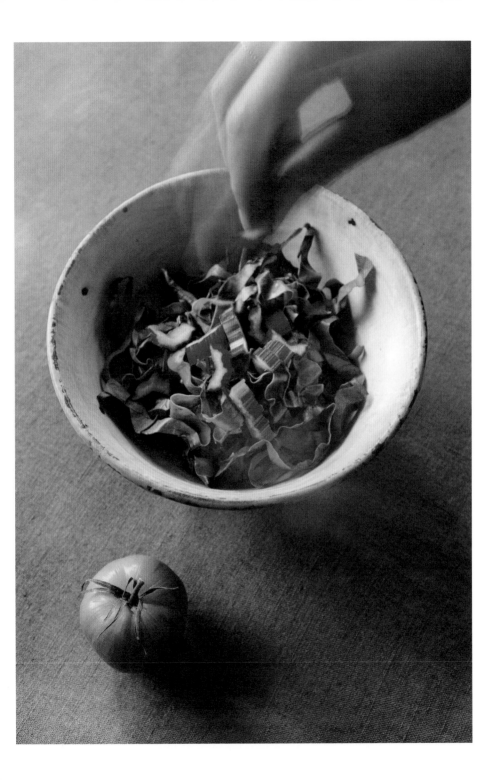

Travel Blast Blessing

This is one of my favourite things to do on public transport: I spread a little sparkle on my journey. Internally I send everyone blessings, blessing their day, their life, their hearts. It's not that I'm doing anything to them, it's more like I'm wishing all parts of their life well.

◎ While on the train or bus or walking down the road, send anyone and everyone you see blessings.

◎ Bless their health, their wealth, their lives, their hearts.

Walking Victorious

Sometimes when I'm walking down the street, I feel I need a little extra energy or a top-me-up – I want to bring a bit of pizzazz into my walk. So I do this practice. Yes, everyone looks at me, but it totally perks up my mood and brings extra energy and vibrancy into my heart centre. You could also do this in the privacy of your own home.

◎ Raise your arms in the air in a V shape, breathe into your heart centre and keep on walking. Notice how you feel.

Evening Clearing Candlelight Ritual

Often by the time we get into bed we are exhausted from the day: so much has gone on around us. It's great to clear the energy from the day so that we have a peaceful sleep. Think of this as energy hygiene, similar to brushing your teeth at the end of the day.

Ingredients

candle, matches

◎ Light a candle. Soften your gaze and look into the flame.

◎ Begin by communing with the energy of the fire, saying something like:

"Sacred Fire, thank you for transmuting any dense energies from my day that I no longer need. I offer them to you and I thank you for filling me with your replenishing light."

◎ Close your eyes and sense the energy of the fire coming into your being. Rest in this space for as long as feels good, then when you have a sense that the fire is complete, thank the fire, blow out the candle and enjoy a restful night's sleep.

Calling Yourself Home Before Sleep

During the day most of us interact with many people: we are on the computer, on the phone, communicating with friends, family, colleagues. We are on output – all our energy is going outward.

This is a beautiful ritual for when you get into bed at night. Imagine that you are calling back all the threads of energy you have sent out during the day.

◎ Lying down, hold your hands up in the air so that your arms are at right-angles to your body. Bend your elbows and turn your palms to face you.

◎ Say out loud or internally:

"I call back all threads of energy that I have left with other people, throughout the day, through all my interactions. I ask for my energy to be returned to me."

◎ Feel your energy flooding back into you.

◎ Offer gratitude and drift off into a sweet sleep.

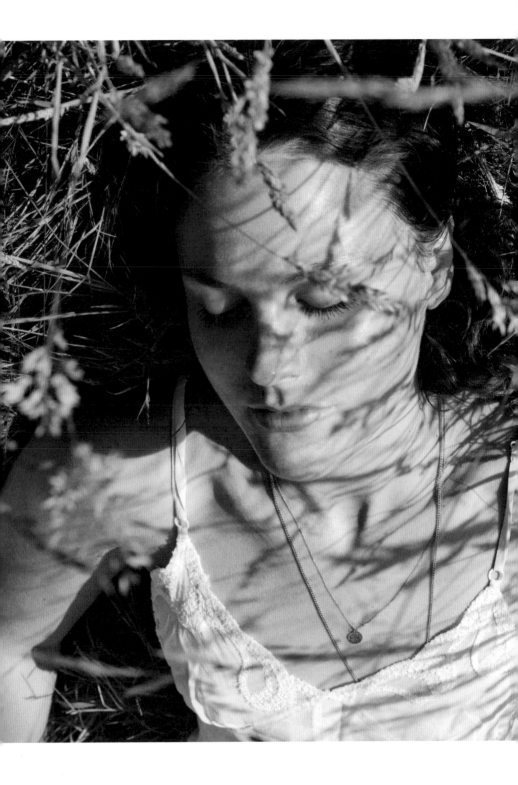

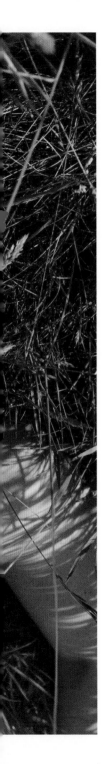

Chapter 3

Sacred Self-love

How do we come into a place of loving ourselves? It's easy to feel good about yourself when you feel great, but what about the days when you just want the world to swallow you up – how do you love yourself then?

For me, learning and practising how to love myself has been the biggest challenge. Growing up, I was my own worst enemy. I had very low self-worth and was constantly comparing myself unfavourably to others.

I knew I had to address this fundamental issue. I went on a quest to learn how to love myself. For me, this is about being tender and kind when I feel dreadful; being gentle with myself when I've not managed to do what I set out to achieve; celebrating myself; taking time to rest and play; listening to and acting on my needs; feeling my Divine presence from within.

This chapter shows the ways that you can bring love and nurturing into your being. When we love ourselves, we emanate and radiate love, spreading it wherever we go. Love creates more love.

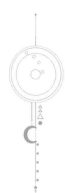

Connecting to Your Heart

The first time my spiritual teacher suggested that I connect to my heart I had no idea what he meant! I was so much in my head, trying to think myself into my heart, that it took me a while to realize that it was about feeling my heart. The first step was becoming aware of how much I existed only in my head, but that I could consciously bring my attention to my heart and tune into my feeling body. This is a powerful ritual to do first thing, when you open your eyes in the morning, and also to begin any meditation.

◎ Place your left hand on your heart or bring your focus to your heart centre.

◎ Send your breath in and out of your heart space.

◎ Drop all of yourself – your attention, your focus – into your heart centre and feel the sensations in your heart.

◎ Rest in this sweet space of stillness. Notice how you feel.

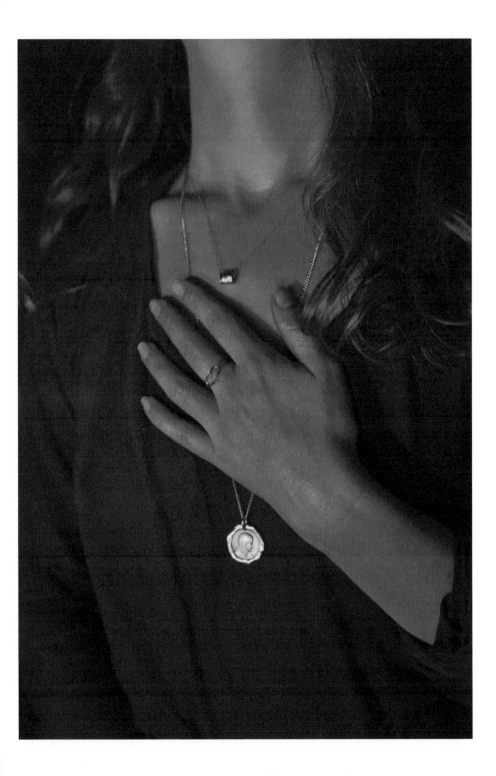

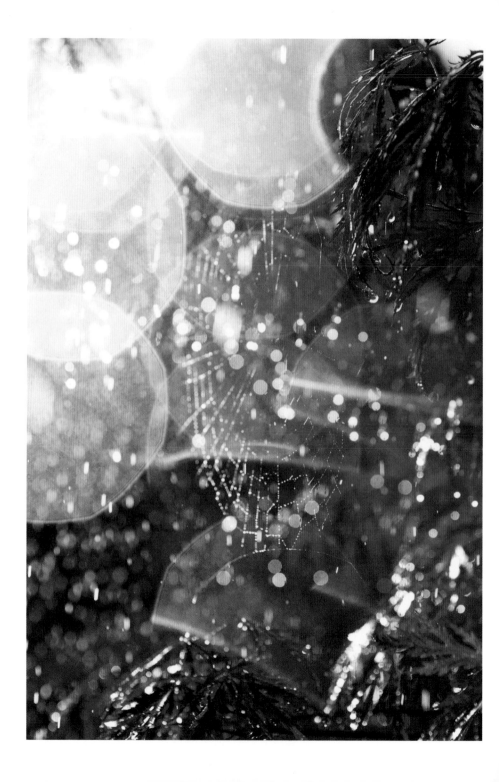

Magic and Miracle Frequency

This is one of my absolute favourites. It can be done any time, anywhere: all you need to tune in and turn on the M & M Frequency is to be grateful. The phrase "M & M Frequency" was taught to me by one of my most adored mentors, Jami Deva, who lives and breathes the Magic and Miracle Frequency and is a shining example of how to truly live in gratitude.

When the idea of gratitude first came into my life, however, the word repelled me! I know it sounds odd, but it's true. Remember that I had spent my teenage years writing depression lists. I realized the reason gratitude repelled me so much was that I was living a life of zero gratitude.

I always remember the day one of my dear friends chimed joyously to me, "Chloe, you're like a holey bucket – anything you put in just falls straight out!" By that she meant that any compliment or good thing that happened in my life, I just could not receive it.

So I went on a quest to mend my "holey bucket" and I found that the only way to patch it up was to be truly grateful.

- ◎ As soon as you wake up in the morning, speak out loud all the things you are grateful for: your bed, your soft pillows, your sheets, your morning cup of tea, whatever you feel grateful for in that moment – it can be anything (see page 36).

- ◎ But you don't just have to do it first thing in the morning. You can be grateful at any time during the day when you want to open up the Magic and Miracle Frequency. It's great for when you feel your mood shifting in a downward spiral – flick the M & M switch and feel yourself come spiralling up again.

- ◎ Notice what happens around you and how you feel when you tune into the Magic and Miracle Frequency.

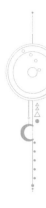

Facing Fears

One of my Shamanic teachers gave me a refrigerator magnet that said, "Everything you want is on the other side of fear." When I first saw it I thought, "Why on earth has she given me this?" Then I realized I was in denial about how much fear was ruling my life. I have learned that when I keep my fears hidden or pretend they don't exist, they become bigger and scarier and take control of my thoughts and behaviour.

Fears that surface in the present, especially when it comes to affairs of the heart, can be rooted in old experiences and patterns that form strong self-beliefs such as "I'm not good enough" or "I'm unlovable". We will often search for external validation to soothe these anxieties rather than give *ourselves* love and compassion, and so when there isn't a constant stream of validation from others, doubts, anxieties and fears creep up on us.

Our response to a fear triggered in the here and now might be an old, well-rehearsed response from as far back as childhood, which explains why you might feel childlike sensations like wanting to hide or cry or be told that it's all going be ok. This is why when I feel fear, I now fully acknowledge my vulnerability, or my "inner child", and ask my inner child what it is they need in order to feel ok.

One time, when I allowed myself to feel into my fear, I sat and cried, allowing the tears to flow, and asked the delicate, tender space inside me, my inner child, "What do you need?" My inner child said, "I need to feel safe."

So I held her in my mind's eye, gently pouring all my love into this delicate part of myself, rocking her, nurturing her, loving her. I said, "You are safe, my love, you are safe." My body softened, my heart relaxed and opened once more.

I knew there was more, so I decided to imagine my fear: the worst-case scenario that my lover no longer wanted me. I was bringing this fear out of my subconscious so that it no longer had a hold over me. I let it be real, bringing the feeling to my heart, allowing it to work through my heart. Then I called on Mama Earth for her support.

The Earth had me, I could feel her power. She was holding me so strongly, I was not alone. Her energy coursed through me all the way to my crown and then to the Cosmos. I was being held by Heaven and Earth, being brought back to my heart again and again and again.

By doing this I was facing my fears, bringing them up into my consciousness so they no longer had a hold on me from my subconscious. This wasn't easy, it wasn't fun and it did not feel good at the time, but in the long run it was worth it. My fears were no longer running the show: they were seen, felt, honoured, and space was given to them.

- ◎ Before you begin, make a choice to feel this fear completely, no matter how painful or scary it is.

- ◎ Call your fear up to the surface of your consciousness. If you're not sure what it is – if it's currently a feeling you can't define – ask to be shown what your fear is.

- ◎ When you know what the fear is, choose to experience it fully. Do not hold back – if you need to, then let yourself cry, scream, howl, whimper or make whatever sound wants to come out.

- ◎ Bring your attention back to your heart; ask for the energy to be moved through your heart.

- ◎ Then ask the delicate tender space inside you, your inner child, what she needs from you. She might tell you that she needs love, that she needs to feel safe or to be heard. Just see what comes up.

- ◎ Once you know what it is, give your inner child whatever she needs. If it's love, love her with all your heart. Imagine holding her, soothing her, speaking words of love to her.

- ◎ There will be a moment when your body softens, and becomes open to receive your own love. When that happens, bathe in it. Feel it, experience it, cherish it, soothing and loving yourself back to wholeness.

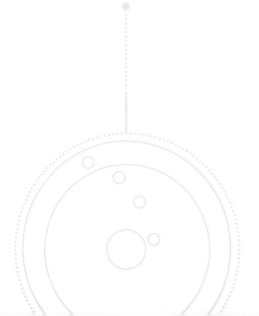

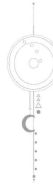

Fiercely Loving Yourself

What if you choose to put your own self-care before anything, to make yourself your number-one priority? Choosing to radically care for yourself, how does that make you feel? I haven't got time? Other people are more important? I don't really know what that means?

I believe that when we choose to look after ourselves, when we choose to love ourselves, we are saying yes to all of ourselves, saying yes to our dreams, our desires and to all of life. Every single person in our life benefits.

Knowing what your core wounds are is the base of sacred self-love and care. Once we know where we are operating from, we have an opportunity to do something about it.

Awareness is the key.

- A situation arises and you feel disempowered. Question yourself: how do I feel? Is it that I don't feel good enough? That I feel abandoned? That I don't feel heard? Dig deep to see what lies at the root.

- When you have your root, allow yourself to feel it completely. It's going to be uncomfortable, it's going to hurt, but it is important to acknowledge and give space to those parts of ourselves that are often squashed down and repressed.

- Ask yourself what you need in the situation. Is it love? Is it to feel safe? To feel heard?

- When you have your answer, ask yourself how. How can I love you? How can I make you feel safe? How can I make you feel heard? Don't think about this for too long: just allow the first thing that occurs to you to come up. It could be the simplest action of giving yourself a hug and holding yourself.

- Consciously choose to take the action that is given to you and do it with all your heart, all your presence and all your love. Choose to nurture, self-care and self-love yourself.

- If tears come, welcome them. The more we welcome all emotions into our life, the more we are accepting all parts of ourselves – the shadow and the light.

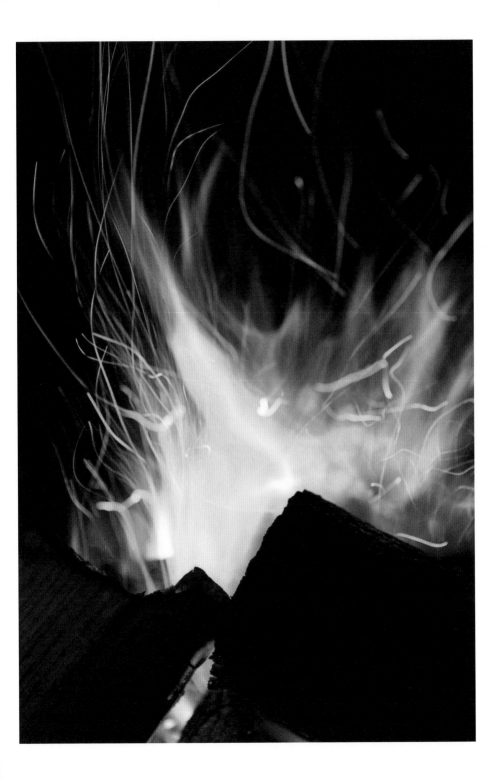

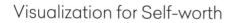

Visualization for Self-worth

Close your eyes, take some deep breaths and come on a journey.

Imagine that you are in a beautiful place in Nature. In front of you, a path forms and leads to a sacred temple. At your own pace, walk toward the temple, noticing that you are carrying a heavy pack on your back. You feel exhausted, weighed down with the load on your back.

As you enter the temple, you are guided by 13 radiant beings to stand in the centre. They surround you, making you feel welcome and safe. You hold out your arms and the beings take off your backpack, telling you that there is no need to carry this heavy weight any more. Breathe a sigh of relief as you let your baggage go. Underneath your clothes you see a radiant blue light shining forth: it is the same as the beings that are surrounding you. You disrobe, seeing that you too are made of light.

Then you hear the Goddess beckoning you. Beneath you a tunnel forms and you head toward the sound of her voice. She says it's time to walk through the fires of creation. She unlocks a door and together you walk through the fire. This fire transmutes old beliefs, old patterns, old ideas, societal beliefs, cultural concepts. See what comes up for clearing. Allow the fire to burn it away with ease and grace, feeling the power of the Goddess beside you.

When you emerge from the fire, you feel the radiant light of the Sun shining down upon you. The sunlight is filled with new codes and frequencies. Feel this light filling you up, starting with your heart and overflowing into every cell of your being. Notice the archangels surrounding you, holding the sacred space. They start singing to you. "You, you are loved, you, you are loved, you, you are loved, you, you are loved, you, you are loved, oh you, you are loved, oh you, you are loved."

You feel yourself being swept away in the bliss of their song, sung especially for you, singing the sound of your heart, your creation song.

A gold triangle forms around you, holding this sacred vibration, solidifying the work that has been done. It is done, it is done.

Thank your teams of light beings, thank the Goddess, thank your angels and thank Mother Father God.

Self-celebration

You may think the idea of self-celebration sounds indulgent – how ingrained is it not to brag and say what an amazing job you have done at something? Well, I think it's time to change that. Time for us to become our own number-one fans, cheering ourselves on. I love having a party for one.

Often out loud I'll congratulate myself, saying, "You're doing such a good job, Chloe", particularly if it is something that I really struggle with. Or if something amazing happens, I'll take time to celebrate. It might be by myself or with others. The important thing is to acknowledge all the amazing things you are doing in your life, no matter how big or small.

◎ Find something to congratulate yourself about, then choose how you want to celebrate yourself. Here are some of the ways you could do it:

- Verbally congratulate yourself by saying, *"I'm doing an amazing job."*

- Do a happy dance.

- Take yourself out for dinner.

- Buy yourself flowers or a present.

- Acknowledge what you have achieved – not playing it down, but celebrating your own success.

- Bake yourself a cake!

Oh, My Love

It's so easy to send love out to others, to love others , but how often do we do it to ourselves? This is a tender practice for consciously giving yourself love.

◎ Place your hand on your heart and say out loud:

"My love, oh, my love."

◎ It's as though you are both the lover and the beloved. Loving yourself just as a beloved would love you. You can look down at your own hands, hold your own heart, seeing and feeling yourself love yourself.

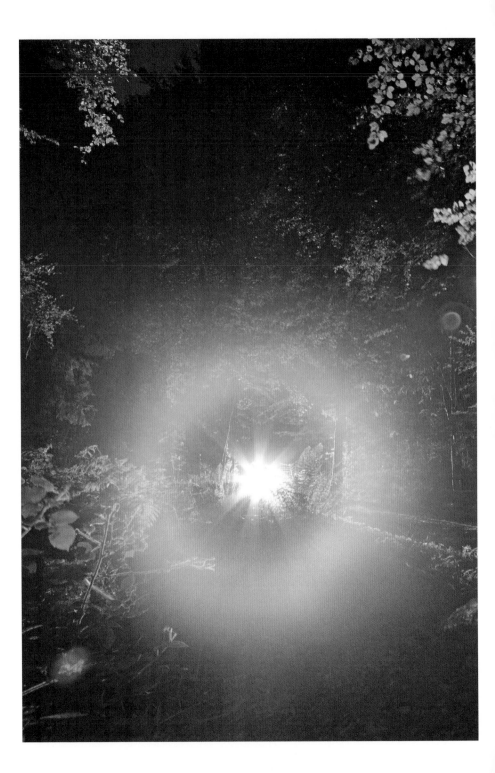

Feeling the Light of Love in Your Heart

Each one of us has a flame of love that burns within our heart. Whether we know it or not, it is there, waiting for us to connect. This flame of love increases every time we bring our attention to it, every time we breathe into it, every time we consciously connect and direct to our heart centre.

◎ Close your eyes, tune inward, take some soothing breaths.

◎ Bring your attention to your heart centre and send your breath in and out of your heart.

◎ Imagine there is a flame in your heart centre and that you are feeding the fire of your heart with every breath. This flame gets bigger.

◎ Can you feel it? Can you rest into the feeling? What do you notice?

Giving and Receiving Love Meditation

Sometimes it's easier to send love to our family members or our pets than it is to ourselves because we naturally love them and want to give them love. This is a beautiful meditation to give the ones dearest to us love and also feel the love for ourselves.

◎ Close your eyes, come into presence and take some soothing breaths.

◎ Imagine someone you have a lot of love for standing in front of you, then send them all of your love.

◎ Imagine a beam of light streaming out from your heart centre into their heart centre.

◎ Imagine another person or a pet, and repeat the practice. Do this three to five times with different people. Feel the love that you are sending out to them, feel your heart giving unconditionally, offering your love.

◎ Then imagine that all the love you are sending out to them turns around in a U shape and all this love is sent back to you, directly into your heart.

◎ Soften and allow yourself to feel and receive your own love. What do you notice?

◎ Give thanks for your heart. Take some breaths and gently come back.

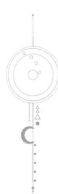

Body Love

I used to be the meanest, cruellest, self-body bully. I had a warped sense of what I looked like and always thought I was the wrong shape, that I was too short, my cheeks were too round, my boobs too small – the list would go on and on and on. One holiday in Glastonbury I had a fall at the foot of a magnificent ancient tree. I twisted my knee so severely that I ended up with a leg splint and on crutches. It was not the holiday I had had in mind: I lay on my back for days, unable to move, and finally, when I could, I was hobbling around on crutches, not even able to carry a cup of tea! The gift in this injury was that it forced me to look at the relationship I had with my body.

Once I couldn't walk, I found a new, far deeper appreciation and love for every part of my body. It was as if I had noticed for the first time what my knees actually do and how much I need both of them! My legs, how they get me around everywhere! My arms, how they were doing all the work supporting me on the crutches. I noticed how many things they pick up, put down, open and close throughout the day. My tummy, my core was actually a loyal friend, the centre of my strength. Thanks to this accident I finally understood and believed that my body is my temple and I really began to feel grateful and appreciate it. I started loving and thanking my thighs, my bum and all the parts of myself that I had previously been so cruel and vicious to!

◎ Move your attention around all parts of your body. Starting at your feet and working your way up the top of your head, give thanks and acknowledge all the things your body has done for you this day. For example, you could say:

"Thank you, my lovely feet, for walking me around all day, taking me here, there and everywhere. Thank you, hands, for picking up my tea, opening the door multiple times..."

◎ Go round all of your body parts, sending them your gratitude.

Salt Bath

An Epsom salt bath is the ultimate relaxation and detoxification. Epsom salt is made up of magnesium and sulphate and it can have many incredible benefits, such as relaxing the muscles and relieving cramps, eliminating harmful toxins, reducing inflammation, improving blood flow and oxygenating the body, improving muscle and nerve function. It's great for joints and skin, too.

Epsom salt is also very supportive for cleansing and clearing your aura, which is the energy field that radiates from your physical body.

I bathe in Epsom salt to cleanse, clear and purify my aura and to relax and rejuvenate my muscles before bed. It always assists me into a deep restful sleep.

Ingredients

candles, matches, 1 cup Epsom salt, essential oils (I like rose, frankincense and lavender: 4–6 drops of each)

- ◎ Light the candles and run the bath, adding Epsom salt and your chosen essential oils.

- ◎ Before you get in, you might like to bless your bath water: place your hands over the bath, connecting to your heart and thanking the water for her cleansing, clearing and purification, sending your love and gratitude, blessing and thanking the water supply all the way back through the pipeline to its original source.

- ◎ Set your intention that this salt bath is for healing and transformation, for releasing and detoxifying any energies from your body that are no longer needed, so that you can open to receive nourishing, healing properties from the minerals and essential oils.

- ◎ Soak and relax for 20–40 minutes.

- ◎ As you let the water out of the bath, imagine all the unwanted energy draining away through the plughole, again thanking the water and offering it to the Earth for transformation.

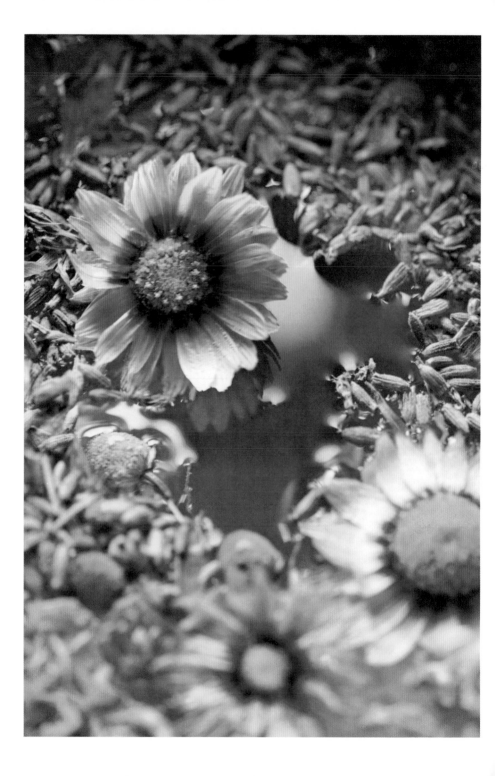

Foot Bath

If we all did this at the end of every day the world would be a very chilled place. It's especially great if you don't have a bath at home. Foot baths soothe, nourish, relax and awaken our whole system. As we know from reflexology, our entire body is connected to our feet – if we nurture our feet, we are caring for our whole body. A foot bath relieves stress and muscle tension and alleviates pain from all parts of the body. It also improves circulation, reduces inflammation, calms the mind and brings the body into blissful tranquillity.

Ingredients

bowl big enough to fit both your feet, handful of Epsom salt or magnesium salt, dried or fresh rose petals, dried or fresh herbs of your choice (I like chamomile, lavender and calendula) and/or essential oils (rose, lavender, frankincense, cedar wood for relaxation; rosemary, clary sage, eucalyptus for clearing – use any oils you feel drawn to and trust your intuition), very warm but not boiling water, towel

◎ Put the salt, herbs and/or essential oils in the bowl, then add the warm water.

◎ Sit in your most comfy chair and place your naked feet in the bowl. Let your feet soak in the herbs and salts.

◎ Relax until the water starts to cool down. Nothing to do, just relax. Dry your feet and gift yourself a loving foot massage (see page 68).

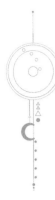

Foot Massage

This is one of my favourite self-care practices because it's so easy and instantly makes you feel good. I do it most nights when I get into bed. If you think about it, our feet are working all through the day, taking us places and being squeezed into shoes. Yet they are the part of our body that we take most for granted and even ignore. Stimulating, rubbing and applying pressure to our feet really helps us relax: it relieves aches and pains, improves blood circulation and assists in a restful night's sleep.

Ingredients

balm (I like coconut oil, almond oil or any other natural oil), your choice of essential oils

- Start with one foot, rubbing in your chosen balm and/or essential oils. Massage your foot, thanking it for walking you around all day, sending it so much love. If you feel a tender spot, gently massage it for a little longer.

- Move on to the other foot: again, give it care and attention, thanking it, sending it love.

- Then both feet together, rubbing, massaging, loving them both. When you feel complete, lie down and feel the tingling energy you have created in your feet.

- Just rest and receive the loving energy you have given yourself.

Sage Bathing

This practice was taught to me by a Sangoma Shaman – a traditional healer from South Africa – at a time when I was highly sensitive and porous to other people's energy. I found that I was picking up on everyone else's feelings and emotions; I might be totally fine and then I would get on the bus and all of a sudden feel low and depressed.

Sage is a natural cleanser, purifier and protector; when you work with plants consciously, it can assist tremendously in strengthening the energy body.

I suggest doing this ritual when you are feeling in need of extra support and strength – I then usually do it three or four days in a row. After I get out of the bath my whole body is vibrating and tingling and I feel much stronger, centred and less porous to outside energies.

Ingredients

4 litres (about 7 pints) water, large pan, a quarter of 1 large white sage bundle (see page 186), sieve

- First prepare the sage water. Put the water in the pan and bring to the boil. Add the sage and simmer for 20 minutes.
- Strain the sage from the water, which will now be a dark purple-brown colour.
- Pour 1 litre (1¾ pints) of the sage water into your bath. Repeat for three or four days in a row with the remaining water.
- Soak in the bath for at least 20 minutes, without adding any soap or salts. Notice how you feel in the sage bath and how your energy field feels when you get out of the water in the coming days. Do you feel more resilient, stronger and protected?
- Once you get out of the bath, give yourself time to relax and receive.

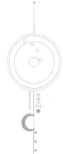

Sacred Sensual Dance

Movement is a powerful way to shift your mood and to move energy. It's also a direct way to bring pleasure into your body. Some mornings I dance because I feel as if I need to move some energy within me; some evenings I dance as I feel filled with sexual energy; some days I dance with my friends for pure joy.

One particular day I woke up feeling very groggy. I knew something had to move, so I put on my sexiest burgundy-red silk dress and started to play my favourite songs. I invited my body to move slowly, sensually, feeling my skin, feeling my curves. Simply enjoying my own body. I noticed by the third song that I was back in my body, on the path of pleasure.

Ingredients

your favourite music

◎ Start slowly, allowing your body to move to your chosen music in whatever way feels good to you. Touch your skin, touch your hair. Dance for as long as you like. Check in with yourself and see how you are feeling – do you notice any shifts?

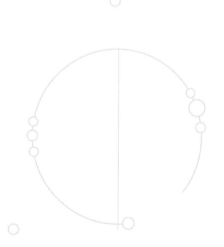

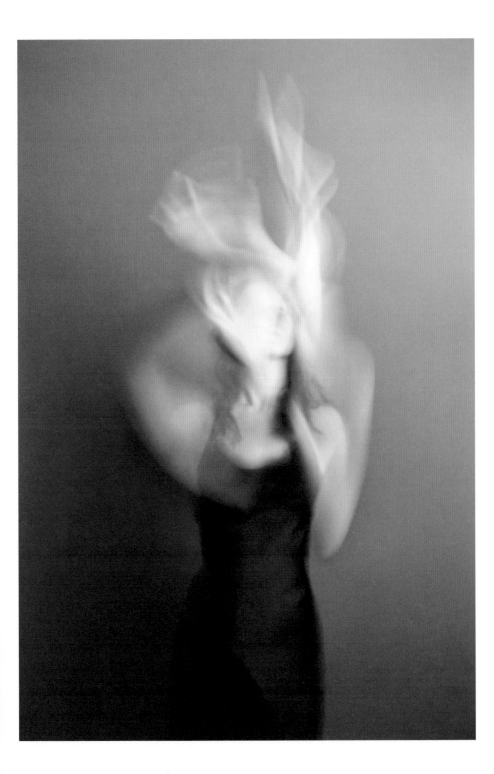

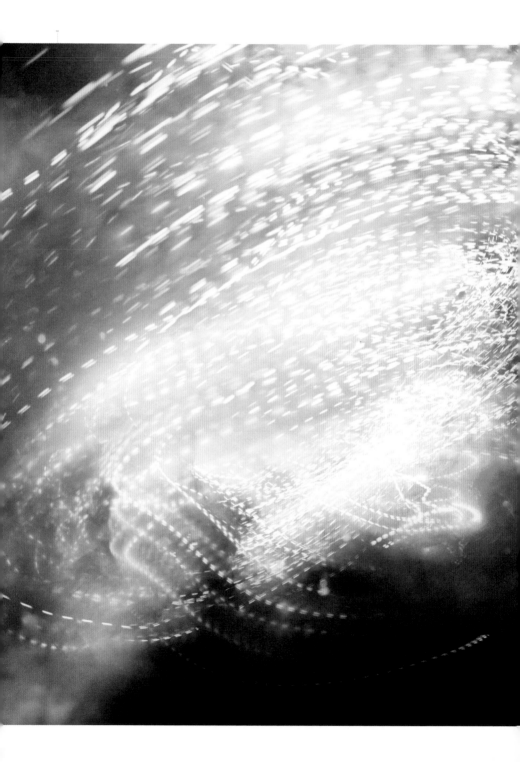

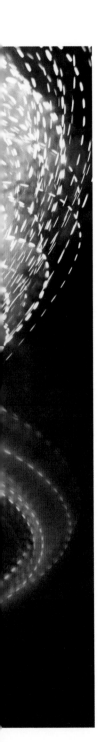

Chapter 4

Affairs of the Heart

Our relationships nurture, nourish and help us to grow. But without self-care, we can become dependent on others for our sense of self-worth or can put aside our own needs for the sake of our partner's.

In this chapter we will explore our inner GPS system and learn to follow our intuition, we will allow ourselves to fully experience our emotions, empower ourselves and love and care for ourselves. We will make ourselves open to receiving gifts of the heart, remembering to return to our Divine Self.

A number of the practices in this chapter are designed to help us through romantic break-ups, but they can also be very supportive at other times of intense emotion or pain. By performing these rituals and practices, we can move through heavier energies and emotions to a happier, lighter experience.

Inner GPS

Modern living has conditioned us to rely heavily on what our mind tells us, when in reality there are many more ways in which we sense situations.

It was such an exciting moment for me when I realized that there were many centres of my body all feeding back different information. My mind, my heart, my inner child (see page 56), my sexual energy and my womb. In one relationship that I had, for example, my mind said, "Do not trust." Yet my heart felt uncontrollable physical sensations of bliss and love. My inner child felt unsafe, rejected, abandoned and uncared for, yet my sexual energy was totally activated and on fire and my womb was tender and sore. Talk about confusing!

What I found so interesting was that all these different parts of me were having such different experiences of the relationship and it was hard to listen to all of them.

I made myself a map and asked my different centres these questions:

"Mind, what do you think? Heart, how do you feel? Inner child, how do you feel? Sexual energy, what are you experiencing? Womb, how do you feel?"

I gathered information from all my centres, which gave me a well-rounded view from all aspects.

⊚ Is there a situation in your life that is causing you confusion or worry? Does the relationship you have with your partner cause you to be unsure or uncertain? Bring the situation to the forefront of your awareness. Ask questions of your different centres:

- *"Mind, what do you think?"*
- *"Heart, how do you feel?"*
- *"Inner child, how do you feel?"*
- *"Sexual energy, what are you experiencing?"*
- *"Womb, how do you feel?"*

⊚ Gather the information. Do you have a full-body yes or are there questions? Do you have inner conflict? If so, look at what the different parts of you are telling you. Think about the triangle of disempowerment (see page 76).

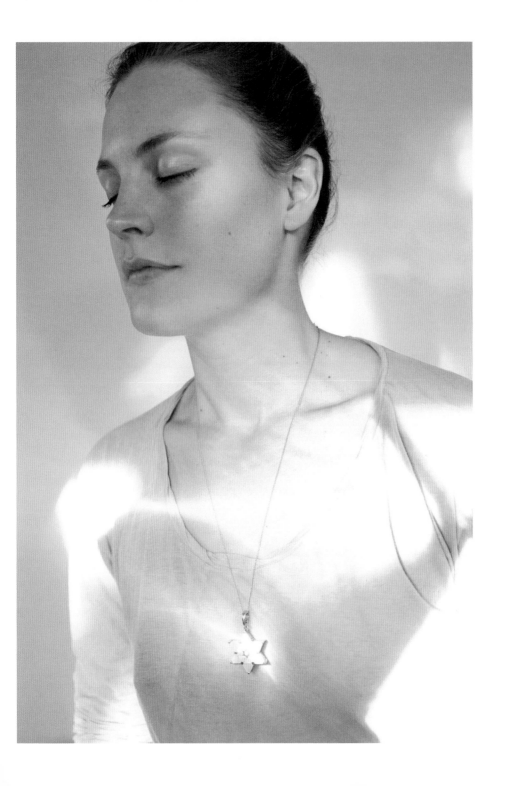

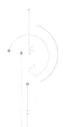

Triangle of Disempowerment

This is one of the most helpful things I learned while studying at the Four Winds Society. It's called the triangle of disempowerment, which is based on the Drama Triangle, originally developed 40 years ago by Stephen Karpman M.D.

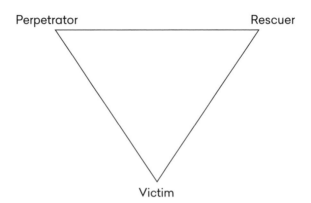

On the triangle of disempowerment sit the victim, the perpetrator and the rescuer. When you are in a situation or conflict with another person, notice if you are falling into any of these disempowerment roles. Are you blaming the other person or acting in a "poor me" victim way? Or are you trying to save the other, fix them, martyring yourself to be the rescuer? Perhaps you are the one who is hurting the other – you are the perpetrator. We often move between these roles, looking for empowerment in all the wrong places, because any time we act from any of these positions, or project these roles onto another, we are standing in the triangle of disempowerment.

But you can step off the triangle of disempowerment, and instead step on to the triangle of empowerment (see opposite). Ask yourself, "How I can love, honour and respect myself in this situation?" As soon as you introduce the energy of self-love, you have the chance to let go of the disempowering roles and choose the most loving and caring course of action.

Triangle of Empowerment

◎ Look at the situation you are in and ask yourself honestly:

"What role am I playing? The victim, the rescuer or the perpetrator?"

◎ Once you have identified the role, ask yourself:

"What benefit am I receiving from playing this role?"

◎ Then ask yourself:

"Would I like to continue this cycle?"

◎ If not, make a choice to step off the triangle of disempowerment on to the triangle of empowerment and ask yourself:

"How can I love, honour and respect myself through this situation?"

◎ Act on the answer you receive.

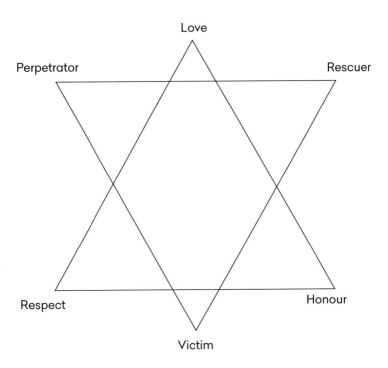

Loving Yourself Through a Break-up

Whether you're the one doing the breaking up or the one being broken up with, it's painful. Even if you both decide, it can hurt. The relationship that you have created together has come to an end. There is naturally a feeling of loss and that often brings grief with it.

I have noticed that after a break-up every day tends to be filled with different emotions. Sometimes it's "thank goodness that's over", the next day a sense of longing and missing, then rejection, anger, rage, deep sadness and grief. It is like being on a rollercoaster, ever changing, up and down, feelings of strength and then hopelessness.

When going through a break-up, every day you can let yourself fully experience whatever emotions you feel. From doing this you can give yourself a newfound strength and feeling of rooted connection to the Divine.

However, you don't need to be going through a break-up in order to do these practices. They can be helpful at any time to move through heavier energy and emotions.

Here are the multiple ways you can nurture and support yourself during the break-up transition, or at other emotional times:

1 Take Every Day As It Comes

How do you feel today? Give yourself full permission to experience and welcome all of your feelings. The more we bottle emotions, the worse and more explosive we become.

◎ Ask yourself some questions. Write the answers down to get the thoughts out of your head.

- *How am I feeling today?*
- *Why am I feeling this way?*
- *What can I do to care for myself in this situation?*
- *What is preventing me from doing this?*
- *How can I honour and love myself today?*

2 The Days That Are Full of Anger and Rage

Rage and anger are powerful energies: if we leave them smouldering in our bodies they can burn us up and cloud even our best relationships. These are also emotions that we often feel ashamed of and so we try to keep a lid on them.

When you feel this rage, I encourage you to embrace it as an opportunity to allow your wild feminine – the part of yourself that is raw and unapologetic – to be exposed. Tap into this energy and allow this part of yourself to roar.

◎ Speak or write all the reasons why you are full of rage. Release all the thoughts that are swirling around your head onto the page or into the ether. Express yourself and acknowledge your feelings.

◎ Dancing is a powerful tonic to stop you stewing and sitting in the rage. Dance it out, put on some rage music, let your body go wild.

◎ Embrace your unapologetic feminine. Find a place in Nature where you can run, punch the air and scream. Give yourself full permission to let your inner wild woman out!

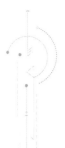

3 Sing Your Heart Out

Singing is another therapeutic way of moving energy. I find that it helps the swirling thoughts to move from my mind and out of my physical body. Before I tried this, I didn't consider myself a musical person, so I was very surprised by the melodies and words that came out of me!

◎ Sing about how you feel or what is around you. One of my first lines was "dragonflies dancing outside my window", because that's what I could see. The next line was "I want to let go but I'm finding it so hard", because that's what I felt.

◎ Play, explore and, if you like what you're singing, record it on a voice note or make a little video on your phone.

4 Support Team

Super-important. Get a couple of your closest, most trusted friends in place, ready for you to call or text day or night, whenever you feel you need support. I would leave voice notes for two of my best girlfriends – I felt so supported, knowing that I wasn't in it alone.

◎ Phone a friend.

5 Nature Nurture

This really is my go-to for everything. Mama Nature is so supportive, she is the ultimate balm. On the days when I felt deep sadness I would curl up on a patch of grass under a tree. Often I would nap and I could feel the Earth draining the sadness from me.

◎ Find a place in Nature where you feel safe and protected. Bring a blanket, curl up and rest. If tears come, let them flow. Offer all your sadness to the Earth. Rest.

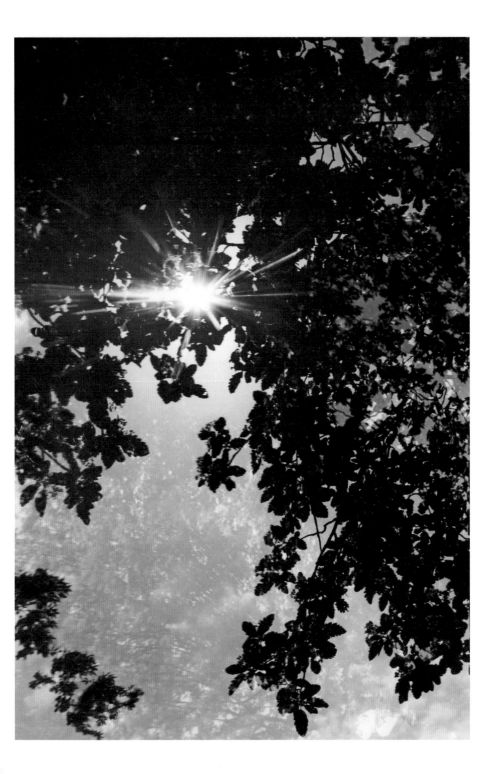

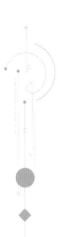

6 The Moments When Your Heart Is Physically in Pain

When my last relationship ended I could physically feel his heart pulling away from mine. It was excruciatingly painful. When the pain began, I felt myself wanting to hold on tight to make it stop.

However, the message I received from Spirit was the complete opposite. It was to soften into the pain instead of holding on and pulling back; it was to fully feel the pain, allowing and inviting my heart to open and feel even more.

◎ When you feel the pain in your heart, close your eyes and take some breaths into your heart centre. Slow down and come into presence.

◎ Imagine that your hand is in front of you, holding tightly on to an object.

◎ Now turn your hand around and open your hand, allow it to let go, stay open and soften. Now physically do this action with your heart. Feel your heart holding on, feel the pain, move toward the pain, invite your heart to soften and open, feeling everything. Rest in this place. Resistance is what causes us more suffering. When we are open and receptive, the sensations can move and healing can occur.

7 Asking for Help from Spirit

On an energetic level we are often still connected to our past partner, but there are many different ways to release these connections. Here's one supportive way in which I like to return to my own energy field.

What happens to me is that I will notice that I'm thinking about my past partner a lot, so I'll know that he is still strongly connected to me in my energy. I close my eyes and ask Spirit to show me where we are connected. I might feel a pull in my heart or solar plexus. I then call upon my angels, particularly Archangel Michael (see page 28). I ask for the cord of energy connecting us to be surrounded in a golden orb of light and ask for it to be returned to Source, to be held in unconditional love. I claim my full sovereignty and freedom. I repeat this as many times as I need throughout the day.

◎ Close your eyes, call on Mother Father God and Archangel Michael. Ask to be shown where you are connected to your past partner in your body. Thank Archangel Michael for surrounding the cord of energy in a golden orb of light, offer the golden orb to be returned to Source, Mother Father God. Imagine the space being filled with golden liquid light and claim your full sovereignty.

◎ Repeat as many times as needed.

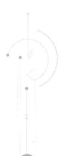

8 Forgiveness

Forgiveness – oomph, it's such a big one and so hard to do! I have had many occasions, particularly when relationships have ended and I felt hurt, when I wanted to forgive and move on, but found it so difficult to actually do so.

I really learned how to forgive after I came in touch with the teachings of Sri Amma Bhagavan at the O&O Academy in southern India, which is a spiritual university centred around awakening humanity. I had come out of a long-term relationship a few months before and I was still holding on to the hurt and blame. No matter how hard I tried with my mind to forgive my ex, the pain was still there – I just couldn't let go. In this particular teaching the monk said that, as your human self, it is impossible to forgive. You can only forgive with the grace of the Divine. Wow, this was huge for me. I realized that in order to truly forgive I had to give it over to God.

- ◎ The first step, as always, is awareness. Acknowledge that you have feelings of hurt toward another person, that you want to let go of these feelings; you want to forgive them but you're finding it hard. Acknowledge that it is impossible for you to forgive in your human form, then call on the assistance of your Divine Spirit.

  "Dear Mother Father God, thank you for helping me forgive … I know it is hard to do by myself. I offer this hurt, this pain to you and I ask that, with your help, I will be able to forgive them."

- ◎ The second step is to ask to see the part that we have played, where we have caused pain to the other person, even when we thought they were causing us pain. Then we ask for forgiveness from them. This can be done internally through meditation or, if it is safe to be in contact with the other person, it can be done externally in person or over the phone.

- ◎ The third step is to ask to forgive yourself for the part that you played and also for the part of you that has not been able to forgive so far.

9 Gratitude

Either we see the bigger picture of why we are grateful for the break-up, what we have learned, how much we have grown, or there might be smaller, more superficial gratitudes for why the two of you are no longer together. Either way, gratitude is the most incredible antidote to pain.

◎ Find even the smallest reasons for being grateful that the relationship is complete. Look for the ways you have grown, developed and what you have learned from the relationship. Send gratitude to all of it.

10 Massage

Part of the great sadness of leaving a relationship is the lack of touch, physical contact, cuddling. I treated myself to massages to make sure that my body still felt loved (see page 96).

11 Self-pleasure

One of the perks of a break-up is the opportunity to have an even more intimate relationship with ourselves. Honestly, we don't need another person in order to make love. At the beginning it might be a bit hard connecting yourself to your own sexual energy, but try it out and keep your juices flowing.

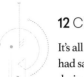

12 Choose

It's all too easy to get into a spiral of thinking about your past partner, wishing that you had said this or that. Or thinking about certain scenarios. This is a complete energy drain and keeps you stuck in negative thought patterns.

Every time I catch myself doing this, I choose to change my thought. I have to be diligent and committed; I have another thought lined up and I switch to thinking about that instead. Or, even better, I bring myself 100 percent into the present moment.

I also ask myself, "What do I choose today?" Here are some of my answers:

- I choose myself.
- I choose my wellbeing.
- I choose my peace of mind.
- I choose to be committed to myself.
- I choose to love, honour and respect myself.
- I choose to come back to the present moment.

◎ Make a commitment to change your thought every time you notice that you are thinking about your ex. Ask yourself what choices you wish to make today and write a list of what you choose.

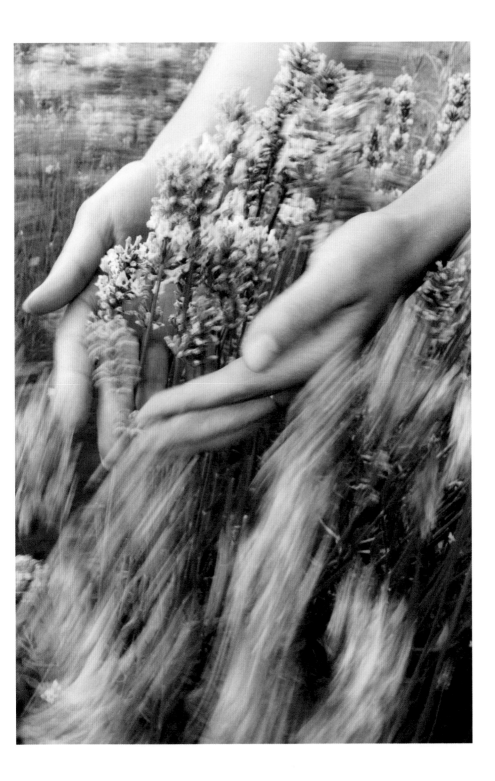

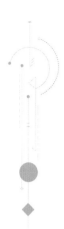

Honouring and Releasing Past Lovers

As I mentioned earlier, when I started on my spiritual path I had been in a three-year relationship. This is a relationship that I found very hard to get over; even when I thought I was over it two years later, it came to the surface during a tantric retreat.

One night I had a dream that my ex was making love to another woman. I woke up in a furious rage that I could not shake off. Even after my shower ritual and scrubbing myself in Himalayan salt, nothing shifted – I was angry. Emotions that I had hidden for years were coming up to the surface and the only thing I could do was feel them.

I knew that Nature would support me, so I took myself off to the woods. While I was there I received an idea to offer an honouring and releasing ceremony. To honour myself, my pains and hurts, to honour the relationship and all that I had learned, to honour all the gifts that I received from no longer being in the relationship and to release it all to Spirit.

I let myself go wild. I cried and cried and cried and then, when I had nothing left to say, I fell on the ground and lay belly-to-belly on the Earth.

I felt the energy drain from me. I could feel the Earth absorbing the energy that I was willing to release. I felt a sense of emptiness and relief. Thanking the Earth, I stood up and received the guidance to find a stone (see page 157).

I walked to the riverbed to look for stones and I couldn't find one anywhere. Then I remembered that I had one of my favourite stones in my pocket. It was so soft, I loved rubbing it between my fingers.

I reached in my pocket, feeling the stone's softness, and I thought, "No, no, no, I'm not going to give this stone away, I'll keep it." In a flash I received a message: "Do you want to hold on to this stone? Just like you want to hold on to the relationship?" As soon as this realization of attachment and not wanting to let go came into my consciousness, I was ready to give my stone away and in turn release the ties of my old lover.

I held the stone up to my mouth and I spoke everything that I was grateful for, every part of the relationship that I honoured, that I had grown from. I spoke of all the joy, all the love, all the precious moments, and I honoured each one of them.

When I was finished and I could think of no more, I took a deep breath and threw my stone with all my might into the river.

As the stone hit the water, I felt what I can only describe as the sensation of a thick rope or a cord being pulled out from the centre of my stomach, from deep within. It was extraordinary, like nothing I had experienced before.

As I walked back to the retreat centre I felt light and clear. I felt that the relationship was complete.

Let me break it down. This is a ceremony to be done alone in Nature.

◎ Set the intention to give yourself full permission to feel and express all of your emotions around the past lover that you are letting go of. No matter if you think you sound like a victim, a weak woman, desperate or angry. Only the trees and Earth will hear you, so go for it.

◎ Express your feelings physically. Move your body in the way that feels right for you – remember you are shifting energy, so be as expressive as you like.

◎ When you feel you have expressed enough, sit – or, like me, lie belly-to-belly – on the Earth, connect with her and notice if you experience energy draining from you. When you sense completion, you're no longer raging and you feel yourself softening, find a stone or a rock and bring forward all the parts of the relationship that you honour: what you learned, the growth you experienced, the gifts that you received together or since you have been apart. Blow them into the stone.

◎ When the stone is filled up with gratitude and honouring, throw it away, preferably into a running river.

◎ Take a few moments to be in stillness and then notice what effect the Honour and Releasing Ceremony has had on you. How do you feel?

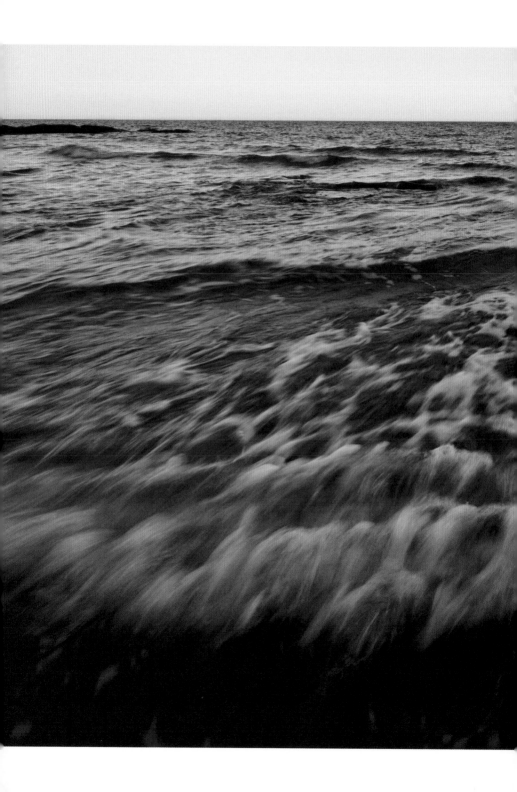

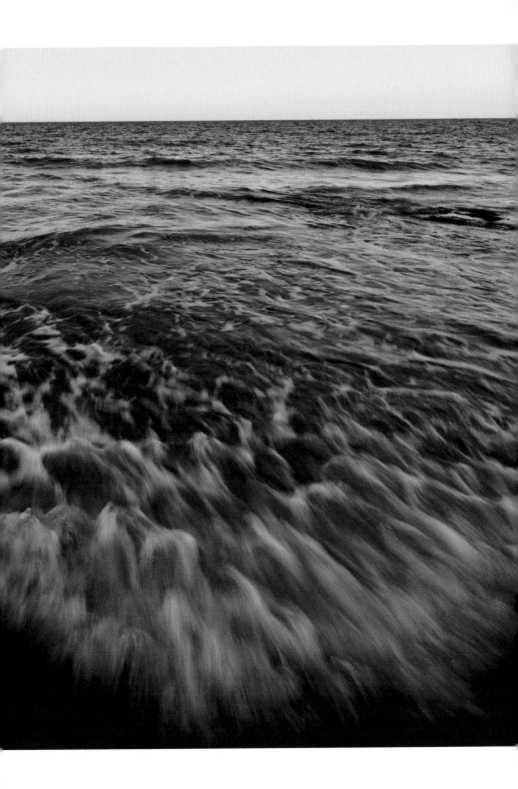

Calling In Your Beloved

Ok, we have got through the break-up, we have empowered ourselves through becoming our own lover and our own beloved. Now what kind of relationship do we want to call into our life from this place of fullness?

Get a laser-sharp focus on what values are important to you, the kind of relationship that you would like to have, and then send the energy out. Remember, in order to attract what you want, you must become what you want!

◎ Get super-clear on the qualities and values you would like to have in a partner.

◎ Write them down in a letter to the Divine. Always start with a thank you, as if you have already received what you are asking for.

◎ Then release it to Spirit, letting go of any attachments, any wishes. Know that your prayer has been heard and so it is.

◎ Ask yourself, *"Am I embodying all of these qualities?"* Remember, like attracts like.

Love Letter to Self

Another beautiful process in becoming your own beloved is to write yourself a love letter. Here's one I wrote to myself.

"Dearest Chloe,

You are doing the best job. I know this is hard for you, but you're doing it, you're letting the relationship go, you're sitting down at your desk, you are writing.

You look so beautiful, your eyes are sparkling, your body is so peachy and rounded.

Oh, my darling, you are so loved, did you know that? You are so supported, you are so held. You are on path, you are on point. You are in your creative flow. Your heart is filled with the Divine Mother's compassion and love.

I love you."

Write yourself a love letter as if you were your own lover. What would you love to receive from someone else?

Keep the letter somewhere safe and, on days when you need to remember how loved you are, take it out to read.

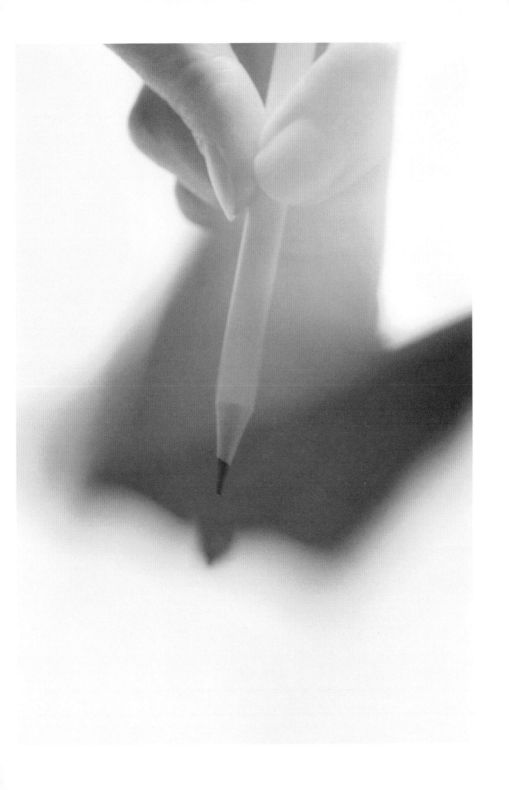

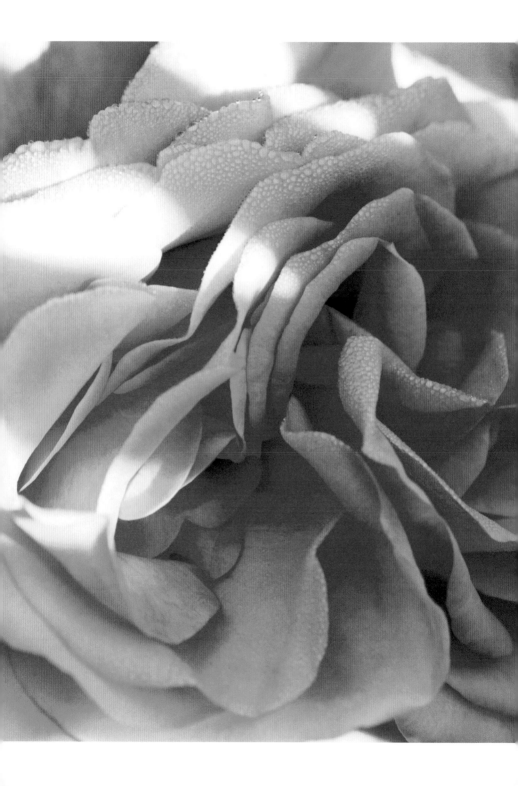

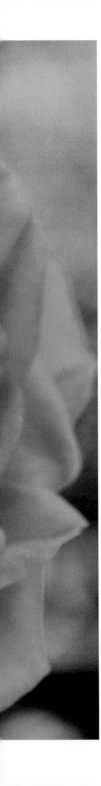

Chapter 5
Feminine Empowerment

Feminine empowerment is incredibly important to me and I bring my attention to it every day. In this chapter we will delve into pleasure practices, menstrual cycle awareness, womb blessings and empowering heart rose meditations. Most of all, we will empower ourselves and celebrate all of our womanhood.

For me, feminine empowerment is about embracing all parts of my femininity and allowing myself to be authentically me, from the sensitive to the wild and raging. It's about being in my body, feeling all my emotions, listening to my inner guidance and following my intuition.

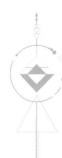

Path of Pleasure

To reclaim our feminine is to connect to all of our sensual pleasure. When we are in our pleasure, we are in our radiance. And so now I like to say that I'm following the pleasure path. By that I mean that I'm constantly looking to see where I can weave pleasurable experiences into my day. It might mean making the most delicious chai or walking extra slowly down the street, so that I can feel my hips moving. Or gently stroking my own skin, feeling the tingles going through my body; smelling an open stargazer lily or sweet-scented rose; or noticing how soft the carpet feels under my toes as I walk up the stairs. The list goes on and on once you start!

◎ Notice in your daily life what brings you pleasure. Is it delicious food? Touching soft things? Dancing slowly? Spending time in Nature? Stretching your body?

◎ See how many pleasurable experiences you can weave into your day.

Walk in Pleasure

◎ Slow your walking down. How does the fabric of your clothes feel on your skin? How does your walk feel? Can you bring in sensual movement and pleasure just for you?

Eat in Pleasure

◎ Slow down and savour every mouthful, taking time to chew. Notice flavours and aromas, smell and taste.

Feel in Pleasure

Self-massage is a beautiful way to bestow love on ourselves. Use coconut oil or another natural oil and your favourite essential oils.

◎ You can begin by stroking your skin. What does it feel like? What parts of you love to be touched lightly? What parts like to be squeezed?

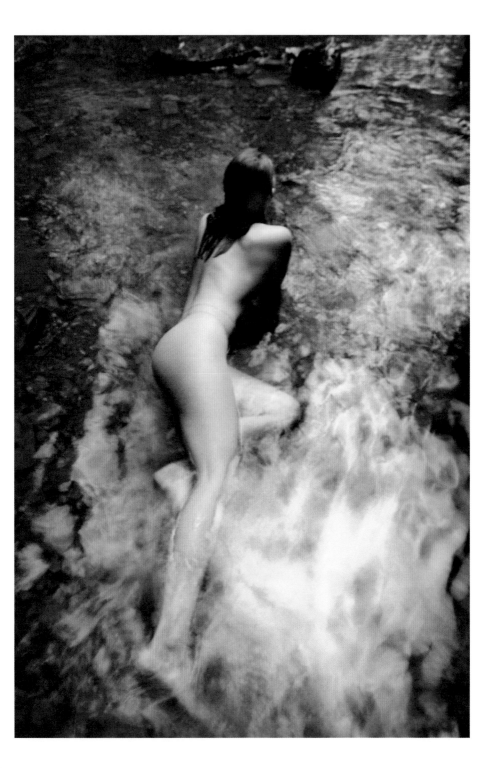

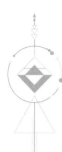

Mirror Me Loving

We are so used to looking in the mirror and only scrutinizing the parts of our bodies that we don't like. But how about making a decision to focus on all the parts that you do like? Look at your eyes, your hair, your skin, the shape of your arms, your bottom. See yourself with fresh eyes. Witness the beauty in yourself. To begin with, it might only be your eyes. If so, just stay looking at your eyes, appreciating them, loving them, adoring them. Every day, spend a little time seeing something that you love.

Date Yourself

I'm so excited and passionate about dating myself! We can so often feel as though we aren't special, that we aren't loved or respected, and people in relationships can sometimes feel that their partner doesn't have time for them. But newsflash: if we don't make time for ourselves, don't respect ourselves, don't love ourselves, how can we expect to attract a partner who will? Like attracts like.

You can date yourself. You can be your own lover and beloved, your own number-one fan, continually filling yourself up, committed to choosing yourself. Loving and caring for yourself in the most impeccable way. And then guess what will happen? You can attract partners who match your loving and caring vibration. It's a win-win!

It doesn't matter if you're single or in a relationship: either way, you can still date yourself.

◎ What would your dream date be? What would you like to eat? Where would you like to go? This could be super-simple or wildly extravagant. Whatever it is, commit to giving it to yourself.

◎ Maybe it's cooking yourself an amazing meal and then taking a long bath; maybe it's going out dancing; maybe it's going to the cinema, out to dinner or to a beautiful place in Nature.

◎ Decide what you want to do and then plan your date. Take yourself out, spoil yourself, love yourself, tell yourself how beautiful you are, enjoy your own company.

◎ Once you have wooed yourself, take yourself to bed and make love to yourself.

Rose Wisdom Meditation

Roses are a symbol of the Divine feminine. They hold infinite wisdom and messages for us. If you look at a rose, you'll see she has a strong, unwavering root firmly grounded in the Earth. Her stem is protected by thorns, so all who approach do so with caution and reverence. Her petals tenderly spiral open with exquisite, delicate and abundant beauty. Her fragrance is hypnotic and her energy magnetic – what is she saying to you?

◎ Sit in front of a rose, soften your gaze and deepen your breath.

◎ How does the rose look to you? What colour is she? What texture are her petals? How is her stem with the thorns? What are the words, feelings and sensations that come to you when you look at this rose?

◎ Close your eyes, soften your body and open to receiving the rose on a deeper, more energetic level. What sensations do you have in your body? What messages does the rose have for you? What knowings do you receive from her?

◎ Write all the words, feelings and emotions you felt on a piece of paper. See your unique rose-wisdom poem form before your eyes.

◎ Offer your gratitude for this connection.

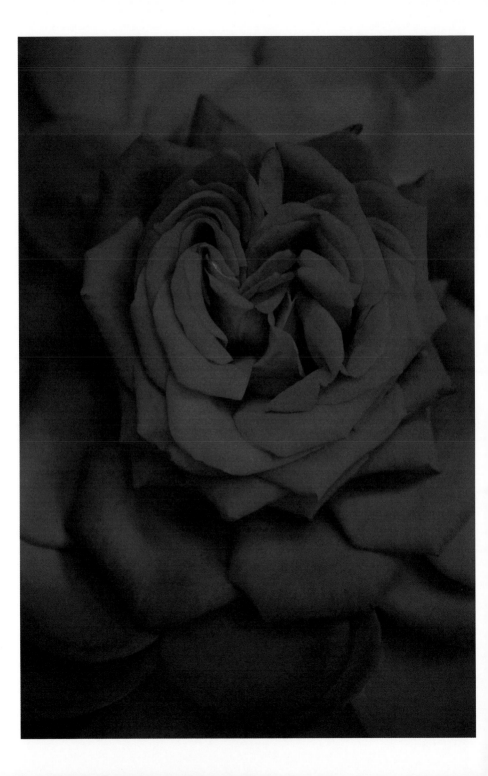

Nourishing Rose Visualization

You can call upon the Divine, loving energy of the rose at any time when you feel you need extra support, protection, clearing and replenishing energy.

- Close your eyes, tune in and take three long, deep breaths.

- Bring your attention to your heart centre. Send your breath in and out of your heart space. Imagine there is a rose growing in the centre of that space. What is this rose like – is it full or limp? Does it have a fragrance?

- Imagine that your rose is deeply rooted in the Earth and ask her what nourishment she would like to receive. Maybe water, maybe sunshine, maybe love, maybe kindness. Be open to how she communicates with you. Once she has told you, drink this nourishment up from the Earth. Notice how your rose changes when she receives this nourishment.

- When your heart rose is in full bloom, tune in to your most heartfelt wish. Imagine that your heart rose is filled with your wish, then send the rose out into the Universe, allowing her to be taken where she needs to go.

- Let the petals fall like blessings for all who need to receive them, then turn your palms upward, allowing a petal to fall into each of your hands. Open to the magic and miracle these prayer petals hold.

- Ask your rose if she has a message for you. Thank her for her love, support and guidance. Take another three long, deep breaths and then gently open your eyes.

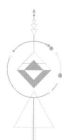

Blessing Your Womb Temple

As well as the heart centre, where we are able to connect with the wisdom of love, women have a second place of wisdom: the womb. It is beautiful to connect the womb and heart centres with this visualization. When we bless our womb space, we are honouring the fact that we and our lives are sacred, and by doing so we acknowledge that all of life is sacred.

◎ Sit or lie comfortably, placing your hands on your womb space, thumbs touching each other, index fingers touching each other to form a triangle.

◎ Bring your focus to your heart centre and then drop your attention to your womb.

◎ Imagine that you are entering into a temple space. Just as you would enter a real-life temple with reverence and respect, sense that you enter your womb temple in the same way.

◎ Give your womb temple an offering. It might be thousands of rose petals, or you might like to light candles, offer blessed water, say a prayer: whatever feels right for you. It is all in your imagination, so you have a limitless supply of what you can give to your womb temple.

◎ Then call on the inner wisdom of your womb and ask if she has a message that she would like to share with you. Be open to how this message comes: it could be a feeling, a knowing, a colour, a sound, a word, an image.

◎ Thank your womb wisdom and gently leave your womb temple, knowing that you can return at any time.

Womb-to-Heart Breath

This practice deepens your heart-to-womb connection, inviting creative life-force energy to flow from your womb to your heart, and unconditional love to flow from your heart to your womb. Although this practice can be done at any time of day, it is a great one to do when you get into bed at night. I find it soothes my system, assisting me to connect inward and receive inner messages. Or it gently guides me into a peaceful night's sleep.

◎ Close your eyes and come into presence with yourself.

◎ Place your left hand on your heart and your right hand on your womb. Take three long, deep breaths.

◎ Bring your focus to your heart centre and breathe into your heart – a long, slow inhale. Exhale long and slowly, sending your breath into your womb space.

◎ Take another long, slow inhale, breathing into your womb, then exhale long and slowly into your heart centre. Keep sending your breath between your heart and your womb. Imagine that your breath is moving in a figure of eight between your hands. What do you notice?

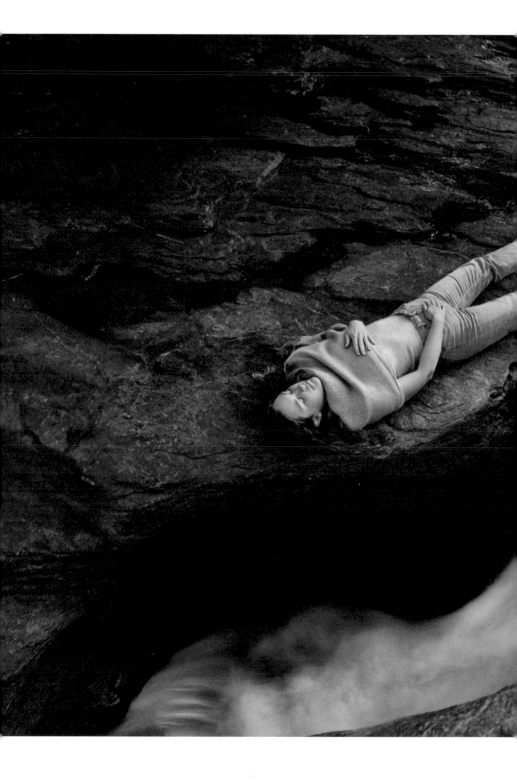

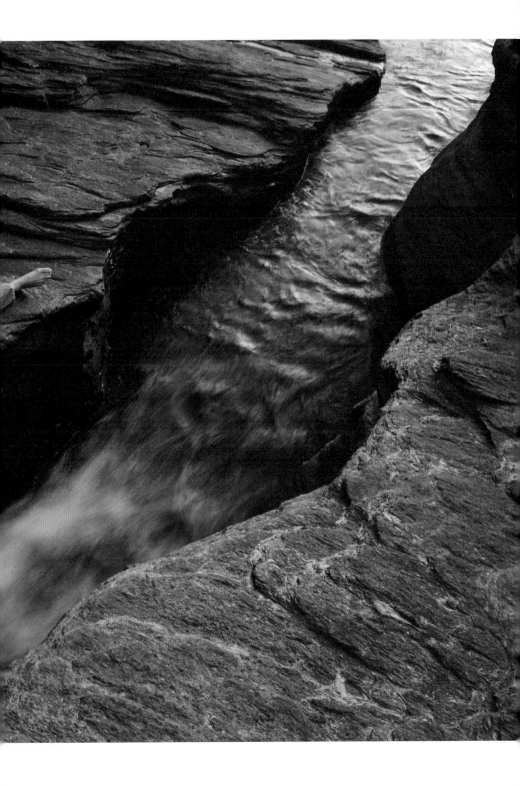

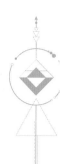

Light of the Womb Meditation

This is a meditation to connect with the light in your womb, and to radiate this light out into the world.

◎ Sit comfortably in a cross-legged position, or lie down if that is more comfortable. Place your hands on your womb, thumbs touching each other, index fingers touching each other to form a triangle (if you practise yoga, you'll know this position as Yoni Mudra).

◎ Take three deep breaths, bringing your attention to your womb space.

◎ Visualize a golden light in the centre of your womb. With every breath, invite your inner womb light to grow. When your womb is filled with light, invite the light to fill up your whole body, from the tips of your toes to the crown of your head.

◎ Allow your light to expand out of your body into the energy field around your body. Feel your light nourish and replenish your whole being.

◎ Tune in and notice any sensations.

◎ Shift your focus to your womb space and ask if she has a message for you. Be open to however the message wants to come: it could be a colour, an image, a feeling, a word.

◎ Invite gratitude to arise. Let this be spontaneous – express thanks for whatever you feel in that moment.

◎ Thank your womb and finish your practice with three deep breaths. Wriggle your fingers and toes and gently come back.

Yoni Love

When I started my womb work, I made a commitment to myself to love, honour and respect my womb and yoni (yoni is the Sanskrit word for vagina and also means sacred temple). One very simple way to do this is by placing your left hand on your heart and your right hand on your yoni. Speak to your yoni, telling her you love, honour and respect her. By doing this you are treating yourself as sacred.

- Close your eyes and come into presence. Take three deep, cleansing breaths.
- Place your left hand on your heart and breathe in and out of your heart centre.
- Place your right hand on your yoni and breathe in and out of your yoni.
- Out loud or internally, speak to your yoni. Tell her that you love, honour and respect her. Tell her that she is sacred.
- Notice the feelings and sensations in your body. Hold your hands in place for as long as you like, then close with gratitude.

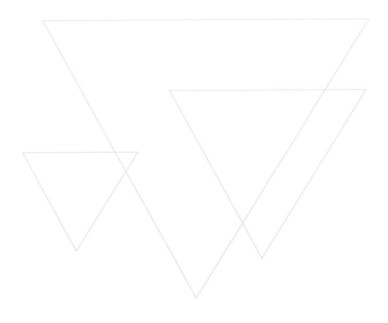

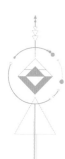

Phases of the Menstrual Cycle

During the phases of life when we are menstruating, we women have an opportunity to discover our personal power and magic through our menstrual cycle. There are four main energies to the cycle – four phases that can be likened to the seasons of the year:

Menstruation – Inner Winter

Pre-Ovulation – Inner Spring

Ovulation – Inner Summer

Pre-Menstruation – Inner Autumn

For women who are not menstruating, the four phases can be connected to the movement of the Moon:

New Moon – Inner Winter

Waxing Moon – Inner Spring

Full Moon – Inner Summer

Waning Moon – Inner Autumn

The following is a brief overview; I strongly suggest reading *Wild Power* by Alexandra Pope and Sjanie Hugo Wurlitzer for an in-depth understanding (see page 188).

Inner Winter: Menstruation

This is the most sacred time of the month, the time when we are most connected to Spirit. If we choose, at this time we can leave the everyday world behind and receive great inner wisdom, insights and visions. We can enter our own inner temple. To be open to this opportunity, we must create time and space to slow down, rest, relax and sleep. Just as our menstrual blood is being released from our bodies, so we can shed and leave the past behind, letting go of the month that has passed since our last bleed.

You can honour this part of your cycle by having some nourishing alone time to focus your energy on yourself. Make space for creativity, draw or paint, play an instrument or write a poem. It's also a great time to keep a dream diary: messages and insights often come to us in our dreams, so keep a notebook by your bed and write down what you dream about.

Inner Spring: Pre-Ovulation

Just like the delicate buds of fresh flowers that grow out of the ground toward the light in springtime, we too can be tender and fresh in the days after we finish bleeding and after we leave the safety of our inner temple. I find there is a sense of newness, playfulness and innocence in the air. From wanting to be internal, all of a sudden I feel that I would like to connect with others again as my energy begins to expand back into the outer world. This is a great time to create space to play, maybe sing or dance. What brings out your playful side?

Inner Summer: Ovulation

Now we are in full bloom. Imagine a rose at her fullest and most fragrant – this is the time when our womb is fertile. It's also when we have the most energy, when we feel as if everything is possible. There is a sense of superwoman powers, magnetism and productivity, and our sensual and sexual energy can be at its most potent. I often have an overwhelming feeling of love for my friends and family at this time – I can give a lot and be there for others. It is the phase of our cycle when we are most connected to the outer world. This can be a great time to schedule meetings, to have a party and to celebrate being you!

Inner Autumn: Pre-Menstruation

And now the harvest has begun, the leaves are falling from the trees. The feeling of being on top of the world, of "I can do anything", often shifts to "What am I doing with my life? Who am I?" This phase can be challenging for some of us: PMS can surface and we become highly self-critical. However, if we know how to love and tend to ourselves, we can see that our cycle is once again supporting us, assisting us to slow down, bringing our focus back inward. It's a time for asking ourselves what our needs are and what changes need to be made. This is a great opportunity to be honest about what you need to address in your life and to take time to be extra loving and tender to yourself.

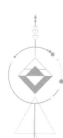

Essential Oils for Menstrual Cycle Support

When I first delved into the phases of the menstrual cycle, it was as if a light bulb was turned on inside me. I always knew I had a part of the month when I felt super-focused and productive, but I didn't know when it was; I had also noticed that there was a time when I experienced a massive dip in energy and questioned where I was going with my life, but I assumed this was just me: I thought I was battling with some kind of depression or low self-esteem that surfaced during the month. I had no idea that it was totally natural and, what's more, necessary for my spiritual growth.

Having learned to love and understand my menstrual cycle, I thought about what I needed to support myself during it and the answer was instantly clear – essential oils. Herbs and plants are so powerful and supportive.

Ingredients

a blend of essential oils (see page 186); I recommend a mixture of the following:
Inner Winter – clary sage, roman chamomile, rose geranium, vetiver
Inner Spring – neroli, bergamot, frankincense
Inner Summer – jasmine, rose otto, sandalwood
Inner Autumn – lavender, rose absolute, clary sage

⊚ Choose the oil relating to the phase of your menstrual cycle and add a drop onto your pulse points (neck, behind your ears, wrists). You could also blend it with a base oil and massge your whole body.

⊚ Repeat the mantra that relates to your menstrual phase (or create your own) as you apply the oils. Add a sparkle of your presence.

Inner Winter: *"I honour myself and surrender to my intuition."*

Inner Spring: *"I embrace my playfulness and respect my innocent tenderness."*

Inner Summer: *"I celebrate my inner and outer beauty, I am radiant."*

Inner Autumn: *"I respect the beauty of transformation, all of me is lovable."*

⊚ Notice how you feel when you open your senses to the oils.

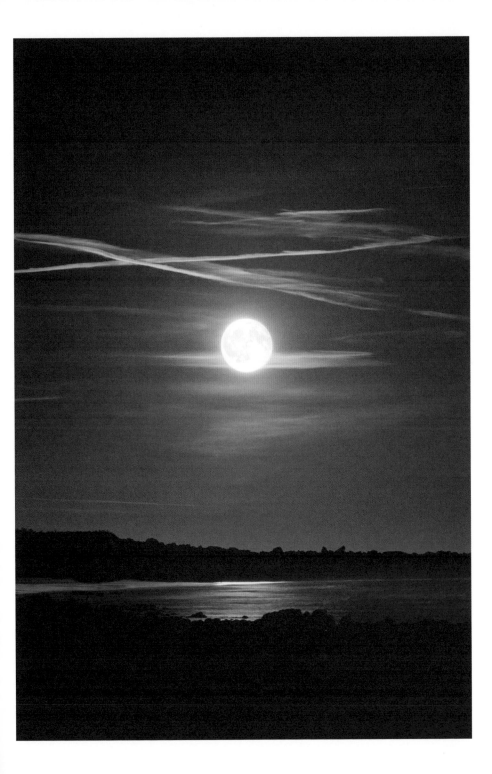

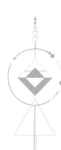

Your Moon Time

One of the highest forms of self-care we can give ourselves is to deeply rest during the time of menstruation.

The first time I really decided to rest on day one of my period, it was quite an experience. To begin with I had waves of anger and rage come to the surface. I let myself feel them; then, once they had passed, I had beautiful, soothing internal messages. The next month I rested again on day one of my bleed – more anger and then very clear visions. By my third bleed, no anger, many visions, messages and then waves of bliss running through my body. A feeling of being totally enveloped in love. Love pouring through every cell of my being: it was ecstatic.

Now every month I give myself space to truly rest and receive while I'm bleeding: it sets me up for the month ahead.

◎ Lie down on your bed or sofa and make yourself comfortable – duvet, pillows, tea by your side. Then just rest. Do absolutely nothing: no reading, no television, no writing. Just close your eyes.

◎ Take as much time as you can, but do try to gift yourself at least an hour.

◎ Notice what guidance is coming to you, but don't do anything about it – just receive. If you want guidance on a particular question, allow your womb and menstrual cycle to answer you. Your intuition is at it clearest during this time.

Moon-time Altar

Another way to honour your bleed time is to create a special altar. When we bleed, it is as though we are entering our own inner temple, a place to rest and renew. Your altar can be the anchor point for this. You could change your everyday altar to a Moon-time one or create a new altar altogether (see page 31 for advice on altar-making).

Ingredients

red flowers and crystals (I like roses and carnelians)

◎ Set the intention that this altar is especially to honour your Moon time, your bleed.

◎ Make the altar with great love. If you have any questions or prayers, write them on a piece of paper and place them on the altar.

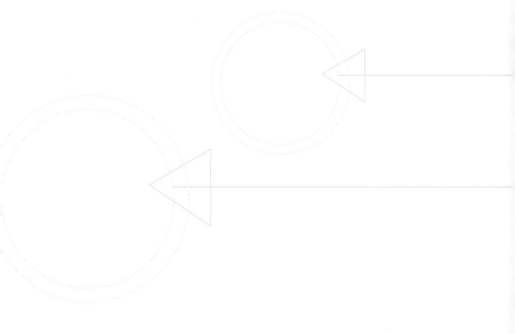

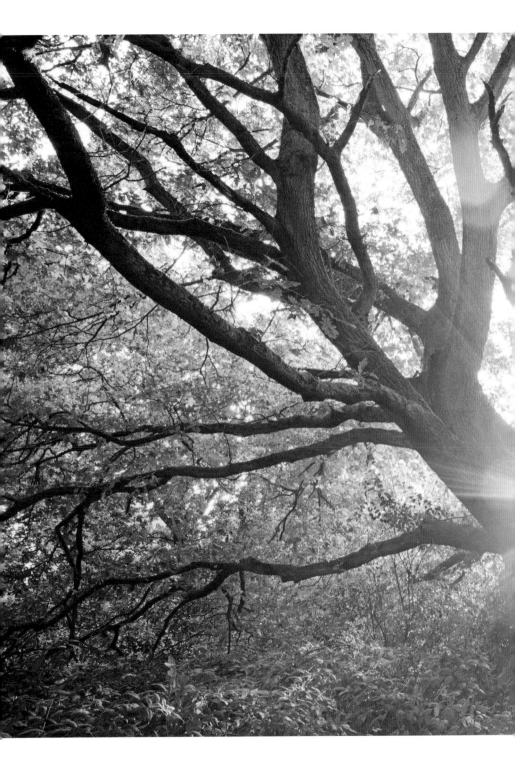

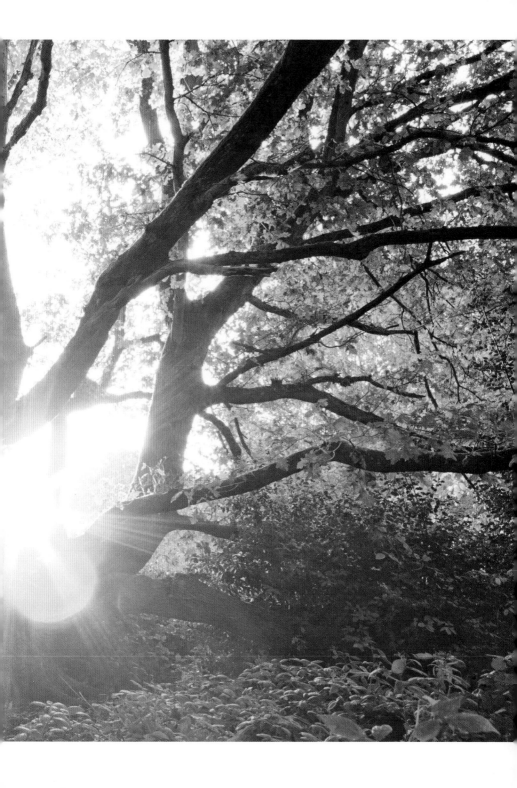

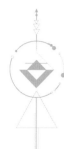

Letting Go When Bleeding

Our cycle can be our most powerful inner spiritual journey and initiation. Every month we get to go through the process of an inner death and rebirth, with the opportunity to rest and receive deep renewal. It is a time to look at the month that has gone by and see what you are ready to let go of and recycle back to the Earth. What are the thoughts, patterns, beliefs and situations that are no longer useful to you? It's a time to identify all these things and consciously choose to let them go with the power of your bleed. A time to identify what you want to release and shed.

◎ With pen and paper nearby, take some time alone. Tune into the month that has passed. What has happened – how have you felt? Look into what you are ready to let go of. It could be a relationship dynamic, a certain situation, limiting beliefs you have about yourself or judgments about others. Take a good internal look at what is going on.

◎ Write down everything you are ready to offer to the Earth, everything that you are ready to let go of, everything that no longer needs to be in your life.

◎ Take your time. Ask to see clearly. Ask to be shown the truth.

Manifesting from the Womb

Once you have done the "letting go" process (see above), you are ready to manifest, which is to call in and create what it is you wish for. Space has been created and the phase of bleeding is a very powerful time to make declarations, to manifest, to bring inner healing and create inner alignment.

◎ Really tune into what you want to manifest this month: break it down into practical, spiritual, heart, for Mama Earth, for humanity.

◎ What are the things that you would like to manifest in your life? They might be career-related, home-related, money-related – what are the actual, physical things?

◎ What are the spiritual? What would you like healing for? What spiritual growth are you praying for?

◎ What are your heart's wishes and desires?

◎ What are your prayers and wishes for our Earth and for humanity?

Moon-time Earth Offering

Alongside the practices of letting go and manifesting from the womb (see opposite), you may like to try offering your blood to the Earth each month. This practice might not be for everyone, but I find it empowering and rejuvenating. You could also use pomegranate juice or red wine.

When we offer our blood to the Earth, in ceremony and with intention, we are honouring menstrual blood as sacred and life-giving; it nourishes the Earth and, by giving it back to her, we are honouring her as well as ourselves. We are acknowledging that our womb and all women's wombs are connected to Mama Earth's womb. I suggest doing the "letting go" process (see opposite) first, in order to be clear about what you want to release and what you want to embrace in the coming month.

I collect my blood using a Moon Cup (see page 186). I then put the blood in a jar – you can keep it in the fridge to stop it from smelling, but it will be fine for a couple of days out of the fridge. When I'm ready (it could be the last day of my bleed or in the middle – I wait until I feel called), I offer my blood to the Earth.

Ingredients

a container with your blood (you can mix water with your blood or just keep it as is) or pomegranate juice or red wine, a place in Nature or a house plant

- ◎ Find a place in Nature where you would like to offer your blood (or you can do this practice just using one of your house plants).

- ◎ Open sacred space (see page 32). Close your eyes. Tune in to what you want to let go: you will already have your list from the "letting go" process, but be open to anything else that might surface.

- ◎ Hold your jar of blood in front of you and speak out loud all the things you are ready to recycle to the Earth.

- ◎ When you feel ready, pour half of the blood into the Earth, with every breath letting go of even more.

- ◎ Then hold your blood in front of you again, and out loud share all the things that you want to create and embrace, your deepest heartfelt prayers for yourself, for humanity and for the Earth.

- ◎ When you feel ready, pour the second half of the blood into the Earth.

- ◎ Now sit or lie down and feel your prayers and wishes being received. Let yourself soften and open to the miracles that are awaiting you. Acknowledge your womb connecting with the womb of the Earth.

- ◎ When you feel complete, close sacred space (see page 32).

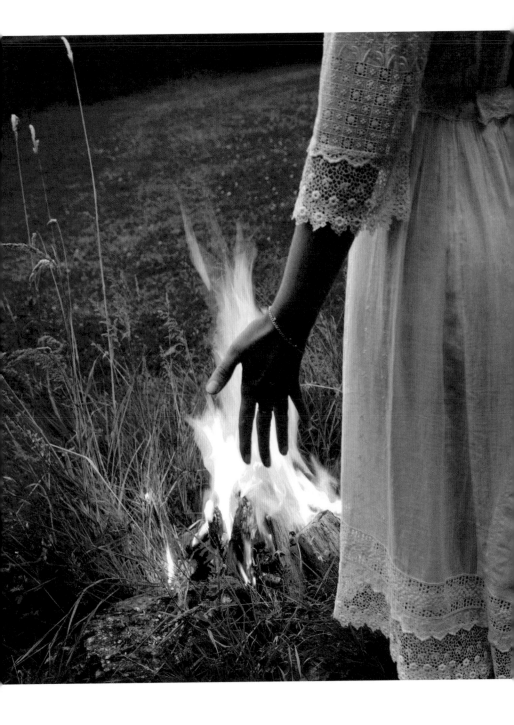

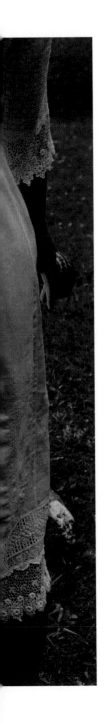

Chapter 6

Sacred Celebrations

For thousands of years tribes and communities have gathered together to celebrate rites of passage, to acknowledge the changing of the seasons, to dance, to sing and to pray together. Sacred celebrations bring people together with a sense of community and connectivity. When we come together in this way, our prayers become magnified and we are embraced in the sacred power that is within all of life. In particular, it is so powerful when women gather together in ceremony.

In this chapter I have suggested ways to harness the energy of the Full Moon and New Moon through ceremony. I've given rites-of-passage celebrations for birthdays, hen blessings and baby blessingway, and shared my most precious devotional cake and chocolate recipes. You can create your own ceremonies by following and trusting your own intuition and inner guidance.

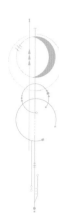

Full Moon Fire Ceremony

The Full Moon is an auspicious time of the lunar cycle to offer ceremony. The Sun and Moon face each other, and the Moon is closest to the Earth. During this time energy is building, there is illumination and an opportunity to expand our awareness. The Moon is at its brightest, amplifying all that is ready to be seen; this can be a powerful time to let go, release, purge. To shed our old, outdated skin like a snake and to offer up personal identities and behaviours that are no longer helpful or supportive in our lives.

This ceremony is based on one I learned at the Four Winds Society, and it is a great way to harness the extra energy and commune with the Full Moon, and open to magical opportunities.

Ingredients

fire pit, two sticks, newspaper, kindling wood, wood logs, drums or rattles (optional), matches, olive oil, sticks that you find (one for each person) to make spirit arrows

◎ This can be done alone or with friends, outside around a fire pit. Before you start making the fire, tune inward, set your intention that this Full Moon Fire Ceremony should heal and transform, aligning your highest destiny or the destiny of others with God's grace.

◎ Make the fire in silence, with full focus and presence. On the floor of the fire pit place two sticks, the first pointing toward the south and the second facing east – this is called a Southern Cross.

◎ Scrunch up pieces of newspaper and place them in the centre, one on top of the other. Add the kindling in the shape of a tepee and finally the logs, keeping the same upward triangle shape.

◎ When you're ready to light the fire, make the commitment that no one will chit-chat until the ceremony is over.

◎ Begin by opening sacred space, calling upon the elements, Earth, water, fire, air and ether (see page 32). It's beautiful if you have instruments such as drums or rattles to play to the fire.

◎ Light the fire and walk around it in a clockwise direction. You're now going to make three olive-oil offerings to the fire.

◎ The first is to the four directions: face south and offer your blessings, then face west, north and east, repeating your blessings, and pour a glug of oil over the fire (this is called feeding the fire).

◎ Next, send your blessings and honourings to the Earth and to the Cosmos, and pour another glug of oil over the fire. Then acknowledge every person in the circle, including yourself, and offer oil to the fire.

◎ Once the flames have settled down and the fire becomes friendly, it's time to make your personal offerings. If you're in a group, one or more of you can approach the fire, while someone else stands behind you with their arms stretched out. They are standing in a supporting role, saying, "I have your back." Approach the fire with great respect – the fire is an alchemical portal of transformation.

◎ You can have all that you would like to release written out on paper, but my preferred way of working is with a stick called a spirit arrow. In one end of the stick you blow and speak all the things that you are letting go, everything that is no longer serving you, all that you want to release, at the same time honouring what they have brought into your life.

◎ When you feel complete, turn the stick around and blow in everything that you want to call in and embrace in your life, blow in your wishes, your dreams for your highest destiny, blow in your prayers for yourself, the Earth and humanity.

◎ When you have finished, throw the stick in the fire (if you have written what you want to release on paper, then throw this on the fire). Thank the fire for her alchemy of transmutation and transformation.

◎ Now, with your hands, scoop up the energy of the fire. Bring this into your womb space, then scoop up more energy and bring it into your heart. Scoop up the energy a third time, bringing it to your third eye (in the centre of your forehead) and letting it wash over your head.

◎ Step back to your place in the circle and allow the next person to come forward. Continue until everyone is done.

◎ With deep gratitude, thank your fire, thank all of the elements and close sacred space (see page 32).

◎ Afterward, sit by the remains of the fire until it is safe to leave it.

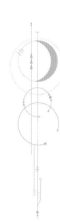

Candlelit Fire Ceremony

Another way to hold a fire ceremony is just with a candle. This can be done simply at home, on your own or with others.

Ingredients

paper, pen or pencil, fireproof bowl, candle, matches

◎ Set your intention and open sacred space (see page 32).

◎ On one side of a piece of paper, write down everything you want to let go and release. On the other side, write down everything you want to call in and embrace in your life, your wishes and dreams.

◎ With a fireproof bowl nearby, burn the paper, honouring what you are offering to the fire, and sending your intentions up to Spirit with no attachment to the outcome.

◎ Thank the fire and close sacred space (see page 32).

New Moon Manifestation Ceremony

When the Moon is new the Earth, Moon and Sun are aligned, and the sky is at its darkest. A New Moon is a symbol of new beginnings, a time to go within yourself, to review and refocus. A time to gather yourself, to reflect on the month that has passed and on what you now want to manifest and embrace into your life.

I find that at the time of the New Moon I'm quite happy to be on my own to really tune inward. I like to set up a little ritual space where I burn candles and incense. I write my New Moon wishes and prayers for the month in my notebook so that I can refer to them at a later date. You will be surprised how quickly some of them come true.

Ingredients

candle and incense (optional), matches, paper, pen or pencil

◎ Light your candle and incense (if using). Close your eyes, turn inward and set your intention.

◎ Write down ten wishes or prayers for yourself, for the Earth, for humanity. Write them in thank-you form, imagining that they have already been granted. Before thanking the New Moon, end your prayers with:

"May the highest good unfold with no attachment."

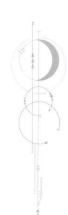

Water Purification and Blessing Ceremony

A water purification ceremony is a time to release, surrender and be reborn. If you think about it, we purify ourselves each time we have a shower or bath, clearing away the day or starting the day afresh. This ceremony is an opportunity to work with Mama Earth's sacred waters, physically and spiritually purifying our body and energy field through the power of our intention, ceremony and water. I have given myself water blessings in rivers, lakes, hot springs and the ocean. They can be done at any time in the Moon cycle.

Ingredients

hand-held crystal singing bowl (optional), rose petals, towel

◎ I prefer to do this practice naked, but if this is not possible or comfortable for you, you could wear a ceremonial dress or even a bikini.

◎ Approach the water with respect. Before you enter it, offer your gratitude, acknowledging that she is sacred, that water is life, that she is the Divine Mother and that her waters are the womb waters of the Earth.

◎ Sing to her. You can begin with sounding *ahhhh*, or see what sounds want to come. Just play – this is an offering to the water from your heart. Maybe words will come and it will turn into a song.

◎ If you have a hand-held singing bowl, it is beautiful to play it. Play to the Nature spirits, to the devas, the fairies.

◎ If you would prefer not to sing, offer your rose petals to the water.

◎ Call upon the elements to open sacred space (see page 32).

◎ When you feel ready, set the intention for sacred waters to cleanse, clear and purify you on a physical and energetic level. You can even say aloud what you intend to release.

◎ Immerse your whole body in the water, including your head.

◎ When you lift your head out of the water, bring your focus and attention to what you are creating and calling to your life, your visions, your dreams, your wishes for yourself, for humanity and for the Earth.

◎ When I'm doing this with friends, we take it in turns to duck underwater. When we rise we call out all that we are embracing in our lives. If you like what your friend has shared, you can say, *"Thank you, bring me more!"*

◎ When you feel ready to come out, imagine that the Goddess of the waters is there holding out a cloak, which she wraps you in. If you can find a spot to sit in stillness, receive the messages the water has for you.

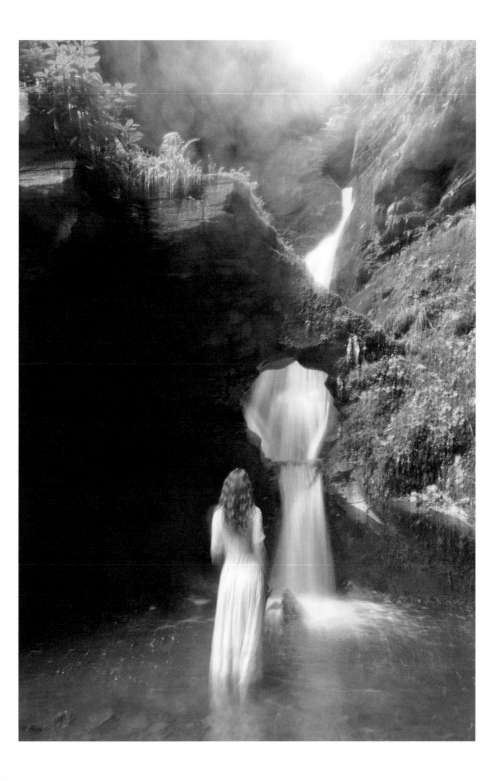

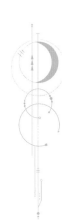

Water Ceremony at Home

This water ceremony is great for when you can't get out into Nature, as it can be done from the comfort of home. It can be done alone or with others.

Ingredients

water (about a small bowl's worth per person), jug, rose water or rose essential oil or another oil of your choice, rose petals or petals from a flower of your choice, water from a place in Nature or sacred site (optional), bowl, ceremonial vessel (this could be a glass, a bowl or a chalice), 1 full rose per person, towel

◎ Wear ceremonial dress or something that you don't mind getting a little wet. You could be naked underneath, or I have done this ceremony naked when I am alone.

◎ Pour the water into a jug. Add a few drops of essential oil or rose water, and your flower petals. If you have access to sacred water, add a few drops to the jug. Bless the water (see page 41).

◎ In a separate bowl, add some more water and decorate with more flower petals. Again, bless the water (see page 41).

◎ Open sacred space (see page 32).

◎ If you are in a group, hold hands, left hand facing upward and right facing down. Drop into silence and presence, taking three deep breaths together.

◎ Sit in a circle and take it in turns to move to the middle, one at a time. The other women are holding a loving, supportive space.

◎ If you are the woman in the centre of the circle, or if you are doing this ceremony alone, pour some of the water from the jug into the ceremonial vessel.

◎ Hold the vessel and either speak out loud all that you are ready to release and offer to the water or silently blow what you would like to release into the water. In a symbolic act of washing this away, pour a little of the water over your head or hands.

◎ Next, speak into the water all your dreams, prayers, loves, your wishes for your highest destiny – again this can be said out loud or blown into the water in silence.

◎ Take your rose and dip it into the blessed water. Anoint your womb, heart, your third eye in the centre of your forehead, and anywhere else on your body (if you wish, this anointing can be done by another woman). Imagine you are being blessed every time the rose touches you, that your prayers are being infused into your being. If there is water left, pour the remainder over your head.

◎ If you are doing this in a group, let each woman take her turn in the centre of the circle.

◎ At the end, take the bowl of blessed water decorated with flower petals. Remove two petals from your anointing rose. Blow your prayers for humanity into one petal, and blow your prayers for the Earth into the other. Place the petals in the bowl of water.

◎ Find a place to pour the contents of the bowl – either into the ground or a body of water. Your prayers and wishes will be absorbed by the Earth and will flow through her sacred waters.

◎ Offer prayers of gratitude and close sacred space (see page 32).

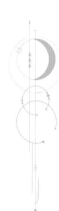

Birthday Blessing

Blessings from the heart are truly a beautiful way to honour a friend's birthday, making them feel seen, appreciated, cherished and adored. Gather together a group of the birthday girl's closest family and friends to perform this wonderful blessing.

Ingredients

a selection of fresh flowers (either picked from Nature or from a florist), beautiful items to create a sacred space (blankets, cushions, flowers, crystals, candles), white sage or palo santo (see page 186) and matches or a celebration blessing spray (see page 27), essential oils, birthday cake or chocolate

◎ If you wish, make a flower crown with some of your fresh flowers.

◎ Before you gather, create a cosy, beautiful space. You might want to move the furniture and make room for you all to sit in a circle on the floor. Or, if it's a fine day, find a spot in Nature under a tree. You could place blankets on the floor or ground and cushions around in a circle; you might want to add flowers, crystals and candles or some other beautiful items. Create a super-special, loving space by putting all of your energy, thought and joy into it, thinking about what your friend would like best.

◎ Add extra magic by burning white sage as you are going around. Thank the sage for her cleansing, clearing and purification of the space. Or perhaps burn some palo santo – this calls in joy and sweetness of life. Alternatively, you could spray a celebration blessing spray (see page 27). As you do this, set the intention to create a sacred, loving birthday blessing and celebration.

◎ When you are all gathered, sit in a circle with the flowers you have collected and your flower crown, if using, in the centre or nearby. Ask everyone to hold hands, right hand facing downward, left hand facing up: this allows the energy to circulate through your circle. All close your eyes and take some deep breaths, dropping into presence with each other. Take a moment just to be silent to feel each other's energy. When you feel ready, squeeze the hands of the friends on either side of you.

◎ See which of you would like to start the blessing and begin by sharing what you love about your friend – what she has brought into your life, why she inspires you and what you appreciate and love about her. At the start, people can feel a little bit uneasy about this sharing, as it's not a natural thing for most of us to do, so it's great to go around the circle twice: by the second time, everyone feels more comfortable and open.

◎ On the second round, pick up the flower crown, if you are using one, and take a flower from the selection in the centre of the circle. This time share all the wishes that you have for the birthday girl and blow these wishes into the flower, then place the flower into the crown. Once everyone has finished, place the crown on the birthday girl's head.

◎ Another beautiful experience is to send love from your heart into her heart. This can be done by sounding *ahhhhhh*, a sound that is directly linked to heart centre.

◎ Ask the birthday girl to sit in the middle of your circle and close her eyes. All together, sound *ahhhhhh*. Keep going and allow the energy to build. Notice what you feel in your own heart.

◎ Imagine white light coming from the centre of your heart and travelling into the centre of her heart every time you sound *ahhhhhh*.

◎ When you all feel complete, gather closely around the birthday girl and ask her what her deepest, most heartfelt birthday wish is. Make her feel super-safe and held as she shares her wishes.

◎ To assist with embodying her wish, ask if she would like a massage or whether she would like to dance or simply sit and talk. If she would like a massage, ask her to lie down in a fetal position. One person can lovingly stroke her hair, another can lovingly massage her back with essential oils, another rub her feet, legs, and so on. Each one of you holds this prayer or wish for her as if it has already come true. Do this for about 10 or 15 minutes; when you feel complete, rest your hands still on her body and sound a final *ahhhhhh*.

◎ Gently help her to sit up again or allow her to rest for as long as she wants.

◎ Bring the blessing to a close by sharing birthday cake or celebrating the birthday girl with chocolate.

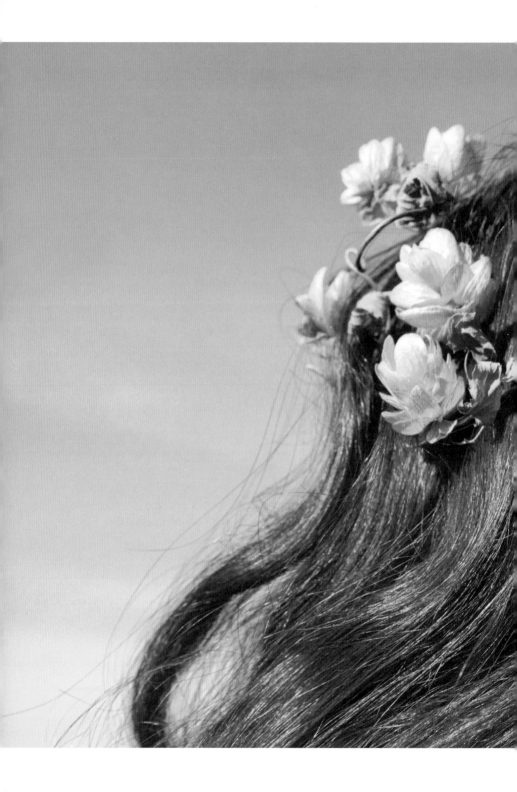

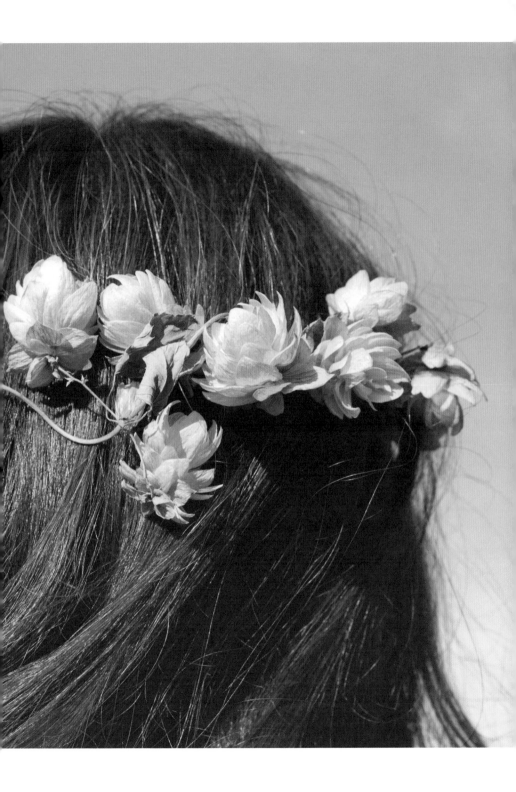

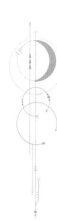

Hen Blessingway

We all know the typical style of hen party and what that involves! I was asked if I could hold a blessing for a hen party instead – the women wanted to celebrate their friend's forthcoming marriage, but not in the "traditional" way. They wanted something beautiful, an experience to be remembered and treasured, so this is what I created. It brings in the elements of cleansing, honouring, celebrating and feasting.

Ingredients

jug, water, rose petals, essential oils (such as rose otto, rose geranium, jasmine or neroli), bowl, small towel, flower crown, fresh flowers (either picked from Nature or bought from a florist, in a variety of sizes: baby's breath, eucalyptus leaves, roses and smaller flowers work really well), sensual music, chocolate

- ◎ Before you start, prepare a jug of water by adding rose petals and essential oils to it. Bless the water (see page 41).

- ◎ Start the blessingway with a meditation to bring you all together. Close your eyes and all hold hands, left hand facing upward and right hand facing down. Take some deep breaths and all focus on your heart centre.

- ◎ One person can lead an opening meditation, such as:

   "We come together to honour and celebrate our dear friend ... for her hen as she transitions into marriage with her beloved. Together we will pour our love, happiness and excitement for the next phase of her life."

- ◎ One by one, take the jug of water and pour some of it over your friend's hands or feet (have a bowl underneath to catch the falling water). This symbolizes a washing-away of what has come before. Pour the water with full presence and honouring for the hen. Dry her hands or feet with the towel.

- ◎ A floral head crown is a beautiful offering. As you pass the crown around the circle, each of you picks up a flower and speaks your blessings and well wishes to the hen – all that you hope for her, all the love that you have for her, why she is so special to you, what you celebrate about her. Blow these into the flower, place it in the crown and pass the crown on to the next sister.

- ◎ Once the circle is complete, place the flower crown on the hen's head.

◎ Now put on some sensual music and play around – dance together, allowing your feminine essence to flow. Enjoy being women together, celebrating another woman.

◎ When you have had enough dancing, sit back down and make a cosy nest for the hen. Each woman can lovingly tend to an area of her body, one massaging her feet, another her hands, back, head and so on. Ask her what she likes and whether you are using the right pressure. Bring all of your nurturing, loving attention to what you are doing.

◎ Then sit in a circle with your hen in the middle. Ask her if she has any prayers or wishes for this next phase of her life. Listen to her and hold a loving space, then imagine that her wishes have come true and make the sound of the heart all together, sending her prayers up to Spirit, *ahhhhhh*.

◎ Close the circle by sharing homemade Raw Rose Chocolate (see page 145).

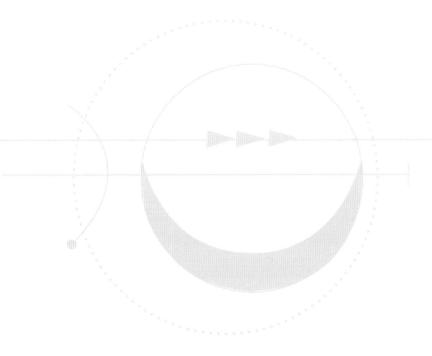

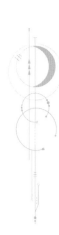

Baby Blessingway

This ceremony is inspired by a traditional Navajo ritual in which women gather together to empower and celebrate a woman's rite of passage into motherhood.

I have attended my cousin's and friends' blessingways and each one was extraordinarily meaningful, tender and sacred. Honouring, nurturing, loving the mama-to-be is the most exquisite way to invite and celebrate the soon-to-be newborn baby into this world.

To create your own blessingway, bring a web of treasured and trusted women together – mother, sisters, cousins, friends, mentors. The blessing assists the mama-to-be in preparing herself for the birth, mentally, emotionally and spiritually, through the love and empowerment of the women in her life, supporting and encouraging her through this incredible rite of passage. By weaving yarn to make an Eye of God, the women come together to create a magical object that can be used as a beautiful baby mobile to watch over and bring blessings to the newborn.

Ingredients

To make the Eye of God: two base sticks, colourful wool to weave (in multiple colours), scissors, talismans (charms and trinkets)

blessing spray (see page 27), water-soluble and pregnancy-safe paints, massage oil, cake and more cake or chocolate, small candles for each woman to take away

◎ Gather in your circle as always, creating a super-cosy, comfy environment (see page 128). Spritz a blessing spray in the air.

◎ This is a time of celebration for the mama-to-be and her unborn babe, it is a welcoming into the Earth. Share the purpose of gathering for the blessingway with the group of women: you are here to share your support, to encourage, love, pamper and empower her into motherhood.

◎ Together, weave an Eye of God. Place two sticks together in an X shape to make the frame. Begin weaving the yarn over and around one stick of the X, then over and around the next stick. Pass the frame around the circle so that each woman does some of the weaving. If you want to change the colour of the yarn as it is passed to the next woman, cut the yarn you are using and tie the next piece to it, then keep weaving.

◎ As each woman takes her turn to weave, she speaks her wishes, blessings and encouragement . Women who have given birth can share birth stories and the mama-to-be can share any concerns she has around the birth.

- When the Eye of God is finished, cut the yarn, leaving a "tail" about 7.5cm (3in) long and thread it through the back to secure it.

- Take the talismans one by one, thread them on to individual pieces of string or yarn and tie them to the Eye of God so that they hang down to create a mobile.

- Then take it in turns to paint a mandala on the mama-to-be's belly if she is comfortable with this. Starting at the belly button, paint shapes, hearts, squiggles, dots – keep going until her belly is fully decorated. This is a time to play and invite creativity to flow!

- Then it's time to nourish and fill her up with overflowing love. Gently massage her shoulders, feet, arms and legs with massage oil, massage her head, pouring all your love into her, making her feel full, loved, honoured, seen and held by her sisters.

- Of course, end with cake and chocolate or eat them throughout the blessing.

- Give each of the women a small candle to take home. When the mama-to-be goes into labour, each woman can light the candle, energetically offering her love and support.

- As always, follow your intuition and allow the ceremony to take shape organically.

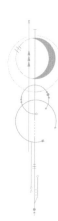

Devotional Cake Rituals

When we make offerings to a deity (a God or Goddess), we are showing our love, gratitude and respect. Offerings can be made in all different ways, from flowers and candles to food and drink – it depends on which deity you are praying to. For instance, if you are praying to a Goddess of Love, you might offer her something sweet and delicious, whereas if you are praying to a Nature Goddess you might offer herbs.

I love to cook in a sacred, ceremonial way. During my time in India, I had many nights when I didn't sleep a wink because the shakti (energy) was so strong, my whole body was vibrating all night. One morning I turned to my friend Callie and said, "Did you sleep?" She replied, "I dreamed I was awake all night, making love to Shiva, making love to Ganesha, to Lakshmi..." The list went on and on.

I knew that I felt I had not slept a wink that night, so I tracked back in my memory to see what I had been up to. And then I remembered, I had dreamed that I had been baking a cake for Shiva, for Lakshmi, for Ganesha and the list went on!

While I do not follow the Hindu religion, I do have a deep love and respect for the deities. And this dream got me thinking about how I could cook for gods and goddesses and turn what I was making into prasad – blessed food.

The first cake I made was for Lakshmi, the Hindu goddess of abundance, prosperity and beauty. I thought that she would like a sensual, rich, dark chocolate cake.

Ingredients

picture of Lakshmi, items that feel sacred to you (such as fresh flowers, crystals or a candle), ingredients and equipment for baking the cake (see opposite)

◎ Begin by creating an altar using a picture of Lakshmi. Place a flower or a crystal on it, or light a candle. Begin with a prayer to invoke her.

"Beloved Goddess Lakshmi, I offer this cake to you, thank you for infusing it with your light, abundance, prosperity. May every person who eats this cake feel your presence and receive your blessings and grace. Deep gratitude."

◎ Play the *Om Shreem Mahalakshmiyei Namaha* mantra on repeat while baking (see page 163). Stay present while you bake, knowing that you are cooking for the goddess of abundance. Tap into your joy and allow Lakshmi to flow through you.

◎ When you cut the cake, offer the first slice to the goddess by placing it on the altar. Offer each friend who is present a slice and say, aloud or inwardly:

"May all your life be filled with abundance, prosperity, beauty and grace."

Mahalalakshmi Cacao Cake

1 teaspoon bicarbonate of soda, a splash of cider vinegar, 150g (5½oz) almond flour, 150g (5½oz) cacao powder, 2 teaspoons ground cinnamon, large pinch of Himalayan salt, 13 Medjool dates, 125ml (4fl oz) hot water, 3 eggs (at room temperature), 2 tablespoons maple syrup (add more if you like it sweeter), 2 tablespoons coconut oil, 2 teaspoons vanilla essence

For the icing

1 x 400g (14oz) can coconut milk (chilled – keep the can in the fridge until needed), seeds from 1 vanilla pod, 2 tablespoons maple syrup

To serve

fresh edible flowers, fresh berries, edible rose petals

- ◎ Preheat the oven to 180°C, 160° fan (350°F), Gas Mark 4. Grease and line a 20cm (8in) round cake tin with baking paper.

- ◎ Mix the bicarbonate of soda with the cider vinegar.

- ◎ In a large bowl, mix together the remaining dry ingredients and add the bicarbonate of soda mixture. Set aside.

- ◎ Place the dates and hot water in a food processor and blend until they form a smooth paste.

- ◎ In a separate bowl, mix the date paste with the eggs, maple syrup, coconut oil and vanilla, and mix until smooth. Add to the dry ingredients and stir until smooth – it should have a consistency similar to brownie mix. Pour the batter into the prepared cake tin.

- ◎ Bake for 25–30 minutes, or until a skewer comes out clean. Leave to cool in the tin.

- ◎ Without shaking the can of coconut milk, open the can and scoop out the thick cream into a large mixing bowl. Beat on high speed with an electric hand mixer until smooth.

- ◎ Slowly add in vanilla and maple syrup and continue beating until fully incorporated and soft peaks form.

- ◎ Once the cake has cooled, cover with the icing and decorate with the berries, flowers and rose petals.

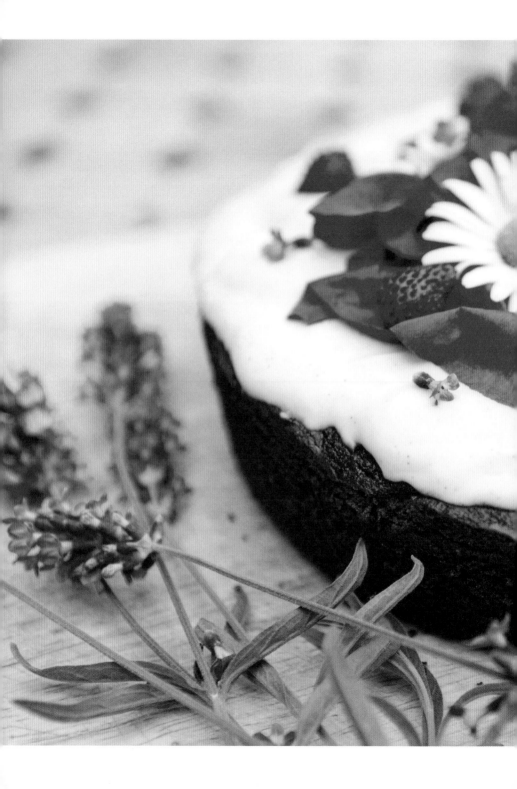

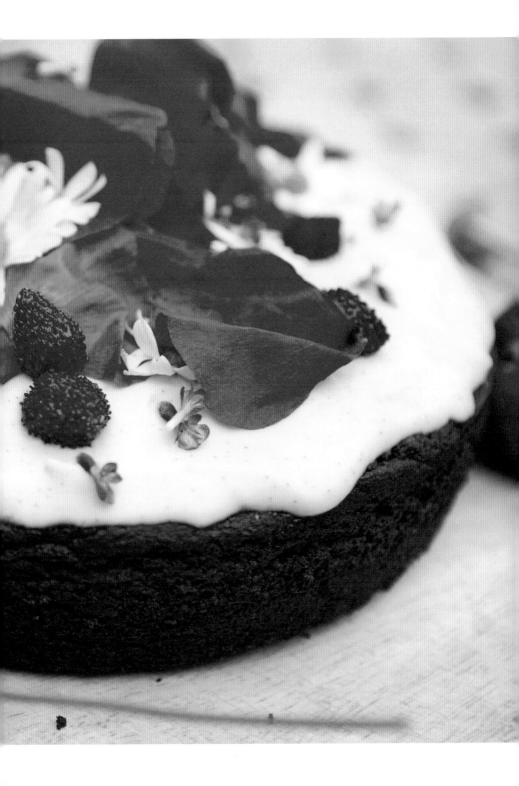

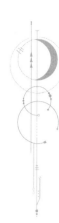

Lord Ganesha Cake

Another of my favourite Hindu deities is Lord Ganesha, who is depicted with a human body and elephant's head. He is known as the master of wisdom and knowledge and as the remover of obstacles in the inner and outer worlds. He represents new beginnings and embodies bliss.

When I was travelling in India I noticed there were often bananas and coconuts on altars honouring Ganesha – supposedly his favourite foods. I created a banana coconut cake to invoke his blessings.

Ingredients

picture of Lord Ganesha, items that feel sacred to you (such as fresh flowers, crystals or a candle), ingredients and equipment for baking the cake (see opposite)

◎ Begin by creating an altar using a picture of Lord Ganesha. Place a flower or a crystal on it, or light a candle. Speak this opening prayer:

"Beloved Lord Ganesha, thank you for removing any obstacles that are holding me back from my highest potential, thank you for opening my path to new beginnings, thank you that I am ready and willing to receive and acknowledge the path that opens up before me. Gratitude."

◎ Put on a chant for Ganesha – *Om Gam Ganapataye Namaha* (see page 163)

◎ Feel the energy of Ganesha all around your joyful cooking, knowing that you are cooking for the Divine, for God, for Source, that you are creating sacred ceremony in your kitchen. You are an alchemist!

◎ Once the cake is cooked, offer the first piece to Lord Ganesha by placing it on his altar.

◎ Offer slices to your friends, outwardly or inwardly saying:

"May all inner and outer obstacles be removed from your path and may new beginnings open with ease and grace."

◎ Notice over the next few days, weeks and month if anything has shifted around the obstacle with which you requested assistance.

Ganesha Banana, Coconut and Cacao Cake

1 teaspoon bicarbonate of soda, a splash of apple cider vinegar, 4 medium-ripe bananas, 4 large eggs (at room temperature), 3 tablespoons date syrup (add more if you like it sweeter), 5 tablespoons coconut oil (melted), 100g (3½oz) gram flour, 100g (3½oz) buckwheat flour, 2 teaspoons ground cinnamon, 1 teaspoon ground cardamom, 1 teaspoon baking powder

For the cacao icing

2 ripe avocados (halved and pitted), 45g (1½oz) unsweetened cocoa powder, 125ml (4fl oz) maple syrup, 2 tablespoons coconut oil (melted), 1 teaspoon vanilla essence, a few pinches of Himalayan salt

For the coconut icing

1 x 400g (14oz) can coconut milk (chilled – keep the can in the fridge until needed), 1 teaspoon vanilla essence, 2 tablespoons maple syrup

For the topping

flakes of desiccated coconut (toasted)

◎ Preheat the oven to 180°C, 160° fan (350°F), Gas Mark 4.

◎ Grease and line two 20cm (8in) cake tins with baking paper.

◎ Mix the bicarbonate of soda with a splash of cider vinegar.

◎ Blend the remaining cake ingredients with the bicarbonate of soda mixture, then pour the batter into the prepared tins. Bake for 45 minutes or until a skewer inserted into the centres comes out clean.

◎ Cool in the tins for 5 minutes, then turn both cakes out onto a wire rack to cool completely. Remove the baking paper and transfer to 2 plates.

◎ For the cacao icing, mash the avocadoes in a bowl then blend in all the remaining ingredients until smooth. Set aside.

◎ Without shaking the can of coconut milk, open the can and scoop out the thick cream into a large mixing bowl. Beat on high speed with an electric hand mixer until smooth.

◎ Slowly add the vanilla essence and maple syrup and continue beating until they are fully incorporated and soft peaks form.

◎ Layer up the cake, with the cacao icing in the centre and the coconut icing on the top. Decorate with the toasted coconut flakes.

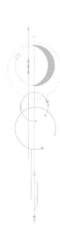

Cacao Ceremony

This beautiful ceremony was gifted to me by my dear friend Louise Shiels from Sound Awakening. Lou is a Cacao ceremonialist and has created this ceremony for me to share with you.

Cacao ceremonies originated in the ancient Mayan and Aztec cultures. Cacao was known as "the food of the gods" and its spirit is thought to be a powerful heart opener and healer, helping you to connect to your inner truth and release old emotional blockages. Cacao is a sacred plant medicine that is non-psychoactive, meaning that it enables a journey of deep self-discovery and brings an opportunity to receive inner guidance. It is high in antioxidants, a source of magnesium, potassium, iron and calcium, and it promotes the bliss chemicals in the body, serotonin, dopamine and anandamide.

I have attended many Cacao ceremonies and each one is very different. I always receive the medicine that I need that day. Sometimes I cry as my heart tenderly opens, shedding past traumas and negative emotions . Other times I dance in overflowing joy or I'm intoxicated in orgasmic bliss. Every time I am powerfully brought to my heart centre and often leave feeling blissed out.

Ingredients

30g (1oz) high-grade ceremonial cacao, 110ml (4 fl oz) filtered or mineral water (add more to achieve preferred consistency), incense, cushions, blankets, candles, saucepan, wooden spoon, cup or mug

◎ A standard ceremonial dose of cacao is 42g (about 1⅓ oz) and this is what most people ingest in a group Cacao Ceremony. With an individual ceremony I prefer to keep the dose a little lower. The quantity I have suggested is enough to really feel the cacao working in you. You can always top it up if you need to, but I find that the longer I work with cacao, the less I need to ingest to feel her full power. Feel free to play around with doses and be aware that if you're caffeine-sensitive (as I am), you may not need as much.

◎ Before you start, make sure you have everything you need. Incense, cushions, blankets and candles are all helpful; I also find that lighting a candle helps call in the higher energies.

◎ Measure out your water into a saucepan and begin to heat it gently. Slice or grate your measure of cacao into the pan and stir gently with a wooden spoon until it takes on a smooth, creamy consistency.

- While stirring the cacao, begin to connect with the plant. Take a deep breath and ask the Cacao Spirit to join you. I like to sing a song, almost like a lullaby, to call in the Spirit, but you can do whatever feels good for you.

- When your liquor is ready, transfer it to a cup or mug. Now you can open sacred space (see page 32).

- Begin by sitting in a comfortable position and taking a few deep breaths to come into your centre. Give yourself permission to relax and to surrender to the experience. Then set an intention for the ceremony: a focused objective helps Cacao to work her magic with you. If you don't have a specific intention, you can simply ask to be open to receive any wisdom, healing or guidance that Cacao may bring.

- With your intention in mind, hold your cup or mug of cacao over your heart centre. Then begin to draw this intention down from your mind and into your heart until you can feel it with your heart. Allow the intention to pour from your heart into the cacao and call on the Spirit of Cacao to be with you and to help you fulfil the intention that you have set.

- Then mindfully drink the cacao while continually pouring your intention into the drink. Be aware of any sensations that may arise as you are drinking and notice how your senses react to the smell and taste. Once you have finished your liquor, send a prayer of thanks to the Cacao Spirit as you begin to feel her warmth and presence in the body.

- Now you can continue to work with her in the way that feels best for you. You might like to try one of these suggestions:

  Dance – dropping down from your head into your body and allowing the medicine to move your body in a way that feels good. See what comes up for you. Become aware of any feelings, emotions or memories. Continue to move in awareness through your dance with Cacao as your guide.

  Meditation – sit in stillness and bring your full awareness into your body. See what arises and passes. What does Cacao bring to your attention in relation to your intention? Sense how the guidance reveals itself.

  Visualization – when you feel ready, lie down and make yourself cosy. Bring your awareness into the body and begin to notice how it is feeling. If you're aware of any areas of tension, take a deep breath and exhale through the mouth, allowing these areas to soften and relax.

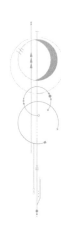

◎ When you feel your body has relaxed, quieten the mind and begin to visualize a place in Nature where you feel peaceful and safe. It can be a place you have visited before or somewhere from your imagination.

◎ Make this place as real as you can, imagining how the air might smell and what sounds you might hear. Then see yourself in this place, seated on a cushion, with an empty cushion opposite you. Invite Cacao to sit with you on the empty cushion. How does she appear? How she reveals herself will be individual to you. Perhaps she appears in feminine form or maybe as a simple glow – remember, there are no right or wrong answers.

◎ Now you have Cacao with you, you can ask her any questions you may have in relation to your intention. With clear awareness, sense how the guidance reveals itself – it is different for everyone. Some people are visual, some hear words and for some it's a deep knowing. Again there is no right or wrong; just be open to whichever ways Cacao communicates her wisdom.

◎ Once you feel you have received what you need, thank Cacao, offer her a big, beautiful hug from your heart and visualize yourself back in your safe place in Nature. Spend some time here.

Raw Rose Chocolates

I am a serious chocolate devotee and to me there is nothing better than making my own. This is my most treasured recipe to date!

Ingredients

100g (3½oz) coconut oil, 100g (3½oz) cacao butter, 90g (3¼oz) cacao powder, 2 tablespoons nut butter (I like almond), 125ml (4fl oz) maple syrup or honey, 2 teaspoons molasses, 1 teaspoon maca, 2 teaspoons cinnamon or edible essential oils (such as rose, geranium, orange, lemon or lavender – see page 186), chocolate moulds

◎ Slowly warm the coconut oil and cacao butter in a saucepan until melted.

◎ Pour into a blender and add all the other ingredients except the essential oils or cinnamon. Blend until smooth and combined.

◎ Mix in the cinnamon, if using. Alternatively, if you are using edible essential oils, decide how many flavours you would like, then divide the chocolate between small bowls and add several drops of oil to each. Taste and add more oil if you want a stronger flavour.

◎ Pour your chocolate mixture into chocolate moulds and place in the fridge or freezer to set.

◎ Then enjoy!

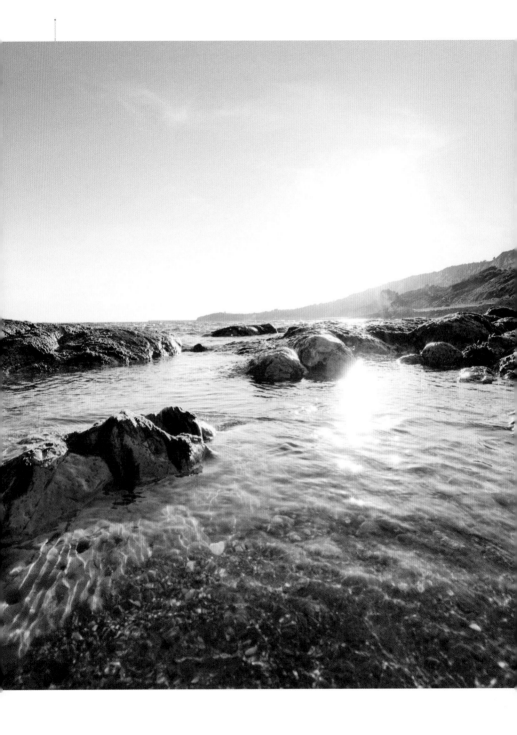

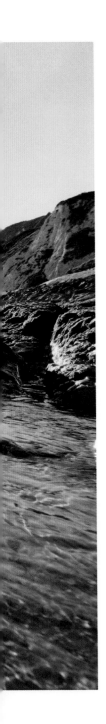

Chapter 7

Staying Connected

It is in quietness and stillness that we have an opportunity to connect and come home to ourself. Time off the phone (that's a big one), time off the computer and time away from other people.

Ironically, in a world of 24/7 digital connection, it is only when we give ourselves permission to rest that we are able to truly connect. In the stillness we open up and become receptive to the messages from within. We connect with the flow of life, with Nature and the beauty in others around us. As we rest, we recharge and then connections come in so many different ways, from a piece of music to singing our hearts out.

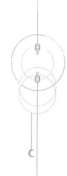

Coming Home to Sweet Stillness

I find the best way to stay connected is so simple, it's almost as if there should be something else with bells and whistles. And yet it is the thing that keeps me the most connected to Source energy, and that is stillness.

The power of stillness and silence is immeasurable. To be still is to connect into the deepest part of yourself, which is pure magic – just focusing inward and resting in this deep, delicious space of pure presence.

From this place, we become self-sourcing and connected to the Divine within. It is simple, yet so powerful. I call it coming home to myself. It can obviously be done any time, anywhere, and we don't need any tools to get there.

- ◎ Close your eyes and set your intention to come home to yourself, to come into stillness. Invite your body to soften and settle.

- ◎ Bring your focus to your heart centre. Send your breath in and out of your heart and rest your attention there. Notice the sensations in your body.

- ◎ Stay here for five minutes or as long as you like.

- ◎ Give gratitude, then gently blink your eyes open and come back.

Charge Up

Truly resting is one of the biggest gifts we can give ourselves: we are often so conditioned to "do, do, do" that resting is something that gets pushed aside.

I like to imagine that we are all human smartphones. Imagine you have been on your phone all day making calls, texting, looking on social media. What happens? The battery runs out.

We are essentially the same: we go to work, talk to lots of people, get on the computer, speak and text on the phone, spend time with family and friends. We run out our inner batteries and often forget to charge ourselves back up again.

The problem is that we are constantly doing things. Have you ever noticed how people tend to ask you what you have been doing, rather than how you are feeling? And let me ask you this. How would it feel to answer, "I've been doing absolutely nothing"? A bit of a conversation-killer! Ha!

The next thing to notice is how resistant we can be to rest. Thoughts are likely to come up that sound like "I should be doing the washing up or laundry or work or calling this person." There are always a million other things that we "could or should" be doing, and taking time to do nothing is the easiest to push to the side.

However, truly resting is deeply restorative. We become more effective, more productive, have higher energy levels and are in a better mood. Sounds good for doing absolutely nothing!

- Start with ten minutes a day when you just lie down with your eyes closed, somewhere super-comfy and cosy. Just rest, do absolutely nothing. If you practise yoga you can be in Savasana pose, or whatever position feels most comfortable. Surrender yourself into relaxation.

- For extra charge-up, this can be done outside in Nature, by a tree on the grass.

- Notice how you feel afterward.

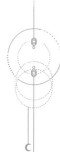

Nature Is the Source

Spending time in Nature is my most-loved spiritual practice. Nature is my temple. When we spend time slowing down with trees, plants, flowers, rocks, rivers, the sea, we become directly plugged into Source energy. Our system reboots and resets, bringing our whole being into balance and harmony.

Whenever I feel wobbly or out of sorts, I know the best place for me is in Nature. If I haven't got access to it, I will find the nearest tree. I physically feel the energy of trees – each one has its own unique quality and feeling.

In 2014, when I went to Peru for the Ayahuasca ceremony (see page 7), one of my prayers was to open and deeply connect to the plant kingdom. After the ceremony I went for a walk and passed by a tree that literally stopped me in my tracks: the vibration coming off it was so strong I could feel it through my whole body. Ever since then I have been able to feel Nature. Just sitting with a tree can give me great relaxation and nourishment.

Once, while contemplating this practice, I asked the plants what happens if other people haven't ingested, or don't want to ingest, Ayahuasca – will they still be able to connect with Nature? If I hadn't, would I have been able to connect? And I received a very clear "yes". Just the wish to connect is enough. It is up to us to make time to sit in Nature, to slow down and receive her energy and her messages.

I love spending time alone in Nature. It makes me feel nourished, held and loved. She is the most exquisite healer. Thank you, Mama Earth.

- ◎ Find a spot that you like the look of and sit down or lie down. Bring a blanket and make sure you are warm enough.

- ◎ Take some breaths and choose to soften your body. Choose to open and receive the Nature around you.

- ◎ Start by listening. What sounds do you hear?

- ◎ Then think about how you are feeling. What do you notice in your body?

- ◎ Allow yourself to drift; let go of trying to do anything and simply surrender yourself to the Earth.

- ◎ Rest here for as long as you like.

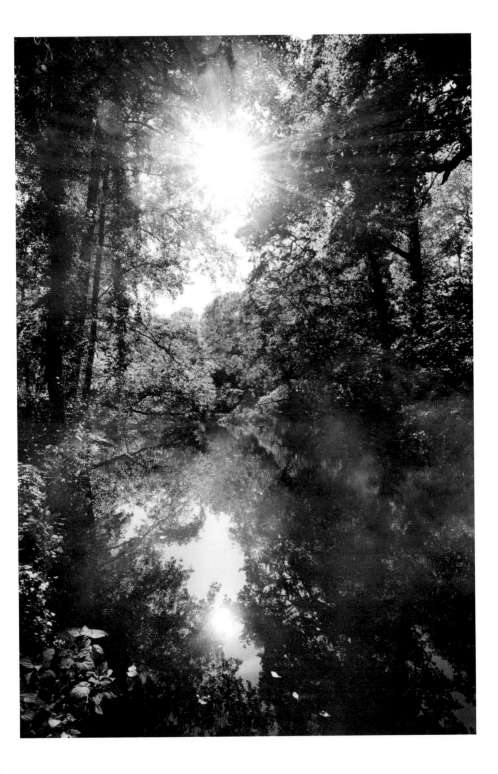

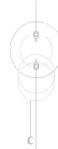

Flower Power

This is one of my most treasured Source connections. I especially like to connect with flowers when I'm in a city and feeling the need for revitalizing energy. If you look around there are often flowers hanging from lamp posts or on outdoor windowsills, or there may be hedges and bushes on the pavement.

I stop at these flowers and hold my hands to them, imagining that they are washing away the sticky city energy and filling me up with radiant, revitalizing light. It works a treat every time. It's an instant refresh and refuel.

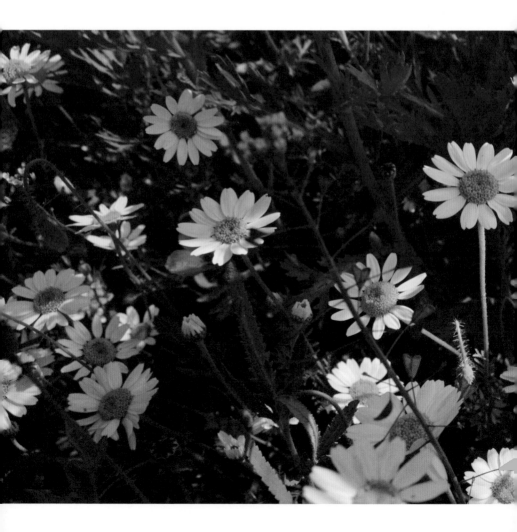

◎ Find a flower, hold your hands up to it, introduce yourself and allow the flower to work its magic on you.

◎ Thank the flower for cleansing and clearing your energy field and for replenishing you with fresh, invigorating energy.

◎ What do you feel? What do you notice? I often find I want to hum *hmmmm* and I feel a buzzing all through my body.

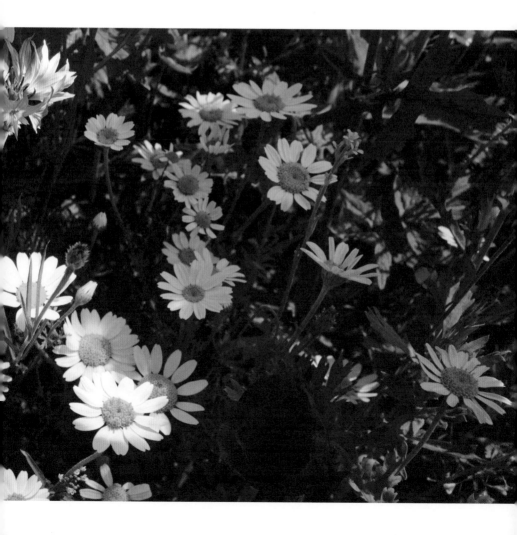

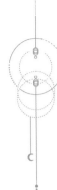

Earthing

Walking barefoot on grass, soil, sand, mud, rocks, any natural surface, is known as earthing or grounding. When we walk barefoot on the Earth we are connecting to the negative electrons that are the Earth's electrical current. Wearing shoes prevents us connecting to this natural charge. Some benefits of walking barefoot and receiving this charge are revitalized energy, restful sleep, a strong immune system and reduced stress.

This is one of the most nourishing and revitalizing practices I do: I feel I am releasing, letting go and recycling energy that is no longer needed back to the Earth and receiving revitalizing, rejuvenating, replenishing energy in its place.

◎ Take off your shoes and socks in a place in Nature or on a patch of grass.

◎ With presence, place your feet on the ground, noticing the feeling under your feet: is it soft and grassy, muddy, wet, dry...?

◎ Slowly walk, noticing every step and every feeling under your feet. Notice how you walk with more caution and take softer steps with no shoes.

◎ Find a place to stop and ask Mama Earth to please take all dense, heavy, unwanted energy from you. Imagine this draining away from the soles of your feet.

◎ Breathe Earth energy up through the soles of your feet and all the way to your heart. Then send it out through your hands, back down to the Earth.

◎ Now breathe Earth energy up from the soles of your feet and all the way to the crown of your head. Imagine the energy going out from the top of your head and circling back down each side of your body, back to Earth. Feel the revitalizing energy travel all the way through your being.

◎ Notice how you feel after this practice.

Tree Time

Ahhh, tree time is incredibly nourishing and supportive. Just by looking at a tree you can tell that it is firmly rooted deep into the ground, its strong, steady trunk unmoving, unwavering, its dancing leaves free to move and blow in the wind. So strong and yet so flexible. Whenever you feel the need for grounding and balancing your emotions, your best friend is a tree.

◎ Find a tree you feel drawn to. Stand with your back to it and take some deep, clearing breaths.

◎ Begin by connecting with the tree: say hello and invite your body to soften and open to receive the tree's medicine. With every breath, notice what you experience in your body and mind.

◎ How do you feel? Do you feel calmer? More relaxed?

◎ You can also start a conversation with the tree: ask what it has to share with you.

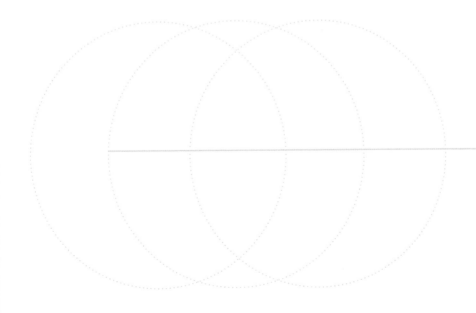

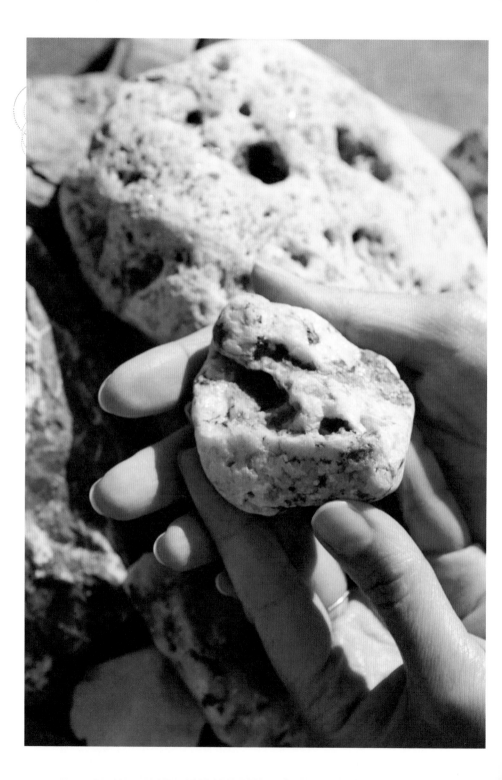

The Rock Speaks

I learned this practice on the very first Shamanic workshop I attended and it has stayed with me ever since. I believe that rocks and stones are living beings with their own spirit, and that they can communicate with us. This practice is a beautiful way to access your intuition through connecting with the stone people. You just need a rock or stone.

Side note: before you take a stone or rock from anywhere, remember to ask if it would like to come with you. I hold the rock in my left hand and ask, "Would you like to come with me?" Sometimes I get flooded with tingles and an expansive feeling through my body, meaning "yes"; other times I feel nothing or I get a firm "no". When that happens, no matter how much I want to take this rock home, I leave it where I found it!

◎ Find a rock, perhaps one you already have asked, and thank it for communing with you.

◎ Have a question in mind. I usually do this practice when something is perplexing me and I just can't find the answer on my own.

◎ Then look at the surface of the rock and see what shapes you notice. It could be a rose, a pyramid, a snake, a diamond. Ask your question to all the shapes you see. For example, the question might be:

"How do I know that I'm following my heart?"

◎ Ask the Rose and you might get the answer, *"Rose says you are following your heart when you feel me open and bloom."*

◎ Pyramid might say, *"You are following your heart when you sink into your ancient inner wisdom."*

◎ Snake says, *"You are following your heart when you allow your layers to shed."*

◎ Diamond says, *"You are following your heart when you express through all the multiple facets of yourself."*

◎ Then create a sentence:

"I am following my heart when I feel myself open and bloom, when I sink into my ancient inner wisdom, when I allow my layers to shed and when I express through all the multiple facets of myself."

◎ Ask any question and allow the rock to speak back to you!

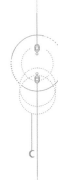

Follow Your Joy

My dear friend and teacher Aravel, whom I mentioned early on, would always say to me, "Follow your joy." After my days in fashion I didn't really know what brought me joy. I was fixated on the idea that joy meant something big. Then I realized I just needed to follow the little things. This created a motion and built momentum: the small joys created more small joys, which then felt like bigger joy!

Flowers make me squeak with joy, making chai mid-morning brings me joy, dancing brings me joy, massaging my body and feet brings me joy, delicious chocolate brings me joy, laughing brings me joy, feeling the soft grass under my bare feet brings me joy.

You see what I mean: they are all so simple, but once you have lots of things that bring you joy, all of a sudden most of your day is filled with joy. Joy creates more joy, just as love creates more love.

◎ Start noticing what brings you joy and do these things often. See how many joyous experiences you can weave into your day.

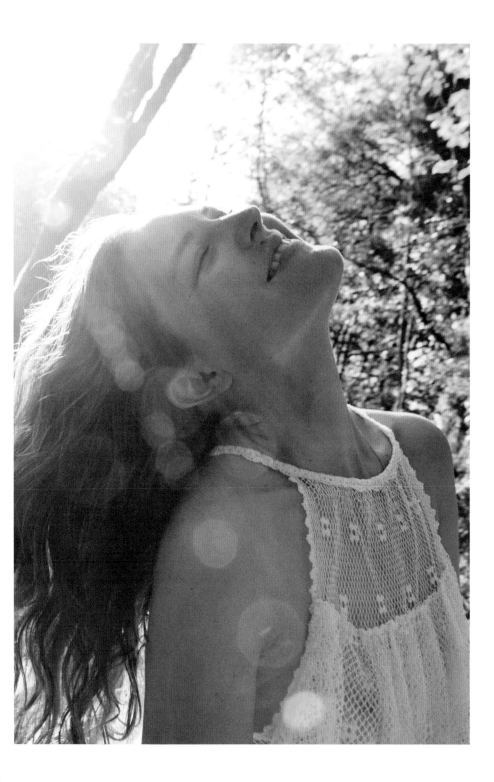

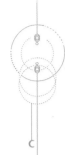

Pure, Innocent Playtime

As children we play all the time, inventing games, allowing our imaginations to take over, but as adults we often forget to play. It's so easy to become too serious about what we are doing.

I remember when I first started on my spiritual path, I became so serious, I didn't want to go to an environment I deemed toxic; I only wanted to have deep conversations. In the process I isolated myself because there were so many things I decided not to do. Of course it's important to be discerning about where you want to put your energy and whether a situation is nourishing for you. But it's just as important to let it all go and play and have fun in the right environment.

Do you know how to play being an adult? It took me a little while to find out. I discovered something that delights my inner child (see page 56) and that I would spend hours doing when I was a child. It's spinning around in circles. I love the feeling, I love the giddiness, it makes me burst out into peals of laughter and shriek with delight all at the same time. It's so childlike and I love it! It can be done in a few seconds and needs nothing. This is one of the ways I play.

◎ Discover what brings out your playful innocence, what delights your inner child. It could be lots of different things such as:

- Playing with animals
- Rock climbing
- Looking for treasures like rocks or shells
- Spinning in circles
- Star jumps
- Making a den
- Having a midnight feast
- Colouring in a colouring book
- Baking cookies

◎ Do something every day that delights your inner child and creates playtime, even if it is just for a couple of minutes.

Paint Play

One of the most therapeutic ways to get out of your head and get connected back in is the simple and childlike act of playing around with paints. I find it incredibly soothing and meditative.

Ingredients

watercolour paints, paintbrushes, glass, water, paper

- ◎ Set aside some time, with no agenda of what you want to paint. Start with a doodle and see what comes out.
- ◎ Play and paint for as long as you like. See what magic you create.
- ◎ As always, notice how you feel afterward.

Musical Play

It's funny how different things open up to you at different times. When I was at school I took singing and guitar lessons, but both my teachers told me I wasn't very good and that I shouldn't continue. This had a lasting effect on me, and for a long time afterward I thought of myself as unmusical.

Then I just started to play around. I bought a singing bowl, a friend gave me a sansula (a little percussion instrument sometimes called a "thumb piano"), then all of a sudden I had an urge to learn the harp. So I started lessons and bought a harp. I just enjoyed playing with the instruments – the sounds and vibrations made me feel good.

Now, most days I spend a bit of time playing one of these instruments. Sometimes I make up little songs that I sing to myself. I find it brings me to a joyous place. I'm not worried if I'm good or not. I'm just playing.

Ingredients

any musical instrument you feel drawn to

- ◎ Play around, make sounds, hum, make up a song.

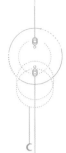

Poems from the Heart

By writing poems, we invite the sweet fragrance of our heart to be shared: expressing from the heart is quite different from expressing from the mind. Our hearts have a tender delicacy that can be shared so beautifully through poetry. Through poetry, you can tune into your heart, letting words flow, not thinking about it too much. Just let your heart speak and feel.

Here is a poem I wrote whilst sitting by a lake watching trees:

"I am the wind that blows in your hair,

I am every breath,

I am the wave, the rippling water's edge,

I am the trees, the leaves and the budding blossom,

I am the stars that light the night and the Moon that shines so bright.

There is nothing that I am not, for I am you and you are me.

Together we will always be.

Remembrance, my friend, is the only key."

◎ Start by writing about what you see and feel. Allow words to flow – don't think about it, just let the words come.

Chanting

Chanting is a very effective way to still your mind, to dissolves worries, fears and blocks and open your heart to connect with the frequency of love.

Chanting repetitively is important if you are to receive the full benefits. With spiritual practice it's best to keep it as regular as possible. It's a bit like going to the gym: you don't go once and expect to get a six-pack, or go to yoga once and expect to do a headstand. You build up your spiritual muscle! Try chanting one mantra for 21 days and see what effects you notice.

Believe it or not, one of my major blocks in life has been writing. So when I began to write this book, I would have an inner challenge that went, "I don't know what to write, I don't know anything. Who am I to write about this? I'm not good enough."

Now, because I know one of my core wounds is a feeling of not being good enough, I can spot this limiting belief immediately. I can do something to change the energy and alter my perspective. So one of my rituals before I sit down to write is chanting.

I chant *Om Gam Ganapataye Namaha,* which is a mantra of Lord Ganesha (see page 140). Before I chant I pray, thanking Lord Ganesha for dissolving all fears and blocks around my writing, for assisting me in coming to a place of openness, believing and trusting that my inner knowledge and wisdom come with ease and grace and are supported by Spirit teams and lineages.

Then I chant the mantra 108 times (108 is considered a sacred number in Hinduism and yoga) and begin writing with a sacred energy buzzing through my body. My mind is soothed and my soul is open to receive Spirit's guidance.

If you are unfamiliar with chanting or have never tried it before, see if there are any chanting circles in your area. Chanting with others is incredibly powerful, as it magnifies the vibration as everyone brings their voices and energy together. There are many different chanting events to try, from a Kirtan (devotional songs usually sung in a call-and-response style) to OM chanting circles, singing circles to drumming circles. Give them a try and see which ones resonate most with you.

Some of my favourite mantras:

Om Gam Ganapataye Namaha *(removing obstacles)*
Om Namah Shivaya *(bowing to inner self)*
Om Mani Padme Hum *(compassion)*
Om Shreem Mahalakshmiyei Namaha *(abundance)*
Om Namo Bhagavate Vasudevaya *(liberation)*

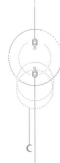

Power of Prayers

To pray it isn't necessary to be religious and I think the word "prayer" often gets a bad rap because a lot of us have had experiences with religion that did not resonate.

However, you may feel there is another guiding force to your life, something that is way bigger than your physical being. I know that the second I embraced that, I felt huge waves of joy and relief. It was as if I knew there was more to life than only what we can see or touch. I had known it as a child, but along the way I forgot or stopped believing. Once I remembered and started having my own experiences, I was in sheer gratitude and wonder. Praying has been a big part of my life ever since.

When we pray we are in connection to the universal consciousness, to Source, Spirit, God, Goddess, to our higher Self, to the unnamable one. For a long time, I felt that my God was outside my Self, but now I feel God's presence within my heart. I feel it particularly when I'm still, when I bring my attention inward.

When we pray, it's to be in gratitude for all that we have and all that we don't have. I like to start with saying thank you. Thank you for my health (without it I can do nothing). Thank you for all the beautiful moments that have happened throughout the day, thank you for all the food I have eaten and water I have drunk. If I'm praying for something in particular, I don't say please, I say thank you, and if the prayer involves someone else, I say thank you that the outcome is the highest for everyone involved. Then I release my prayer to the Universe, almost as if I'm sending up a cloud of smoke, letting go, allowing the outcome to be what it will be.

A friend said to me once, "What is meant for you will not pass you by", so having faith means believing that if something is meant for you, it will come to you. I end my prayer with, "So it is, blessed be." I hold my hands in prayer position to my forehead, for true thinking, then to my heart, honouring the love in my heart; I hold my hands over my womb for wisdom and intuition.

- Tune in, either placing your left hand on your heart or holding your hands in prayer position over your heart centre.

- Focus on your wishes, your prayers, for yourself and also on a collective level, for the Earth and humanity.

- Write or speak (out loud or silently to yourself) your prayers in "thank you" form, imagining that they have already come true. Close your eyes and see your prayers in colour, see that they have already happened and feel how grateful you are.

- Then, and this is the key: let go of the outcome. If other people are involved in your prayer, give thanks that the highest outcome will unfold for all concerned. Imagine that you are sending your prayer to Spirit, letting go of any attachment and any desired outcome. Blessed be, it is done.

- Place your hands in prayer position at your forehead, giving gratitude for clear thought. Move your hands in prayer position over your heart, honouring your loving heart, and over your womb, honouring your source of creativity and life force.

- If the prayer is written, you can place it on your altar for as long as feels right.

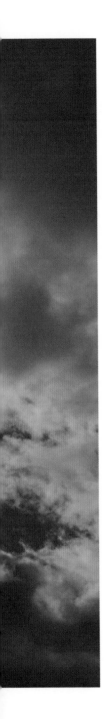

Chapter 8

Emergency

Oh, my goodness. We all know what it is like when we are triggered by a situation and such a flurry of emotions comes up that every self-love and self-care practice seems to fly out the window. Nothing works, and we totally forget all the things that support us. It is easy to fall into a pit of despair. I know this, because I have been there many times.

This chapter is devoted to those moments when you need a hand to pull yourself up, and to remind you of the often very simple ways to connect. It may be calling on your angels for support or opening to receive love from your Earth angels, remembering that you are not alone; resetting fight-or-flight mode; coming home to Nature's temple; or turning on the instant activator of the Magic and Miracle Frequency (see page 55).

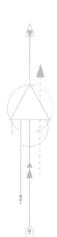

Asking for Help: You Are Not Alone

Remembering that we are not alone is a huge key. Often when we are in a challenging situation, no matter how big or small, we forget to ask for help. When we most need support, we feel the most alone and helpless. When we are overwhelmed and life gets too much, it's all too easy to think, "It's just me."

I was once heading back to London after co-hosting a retreat and I was terribly upset. I felt completely alone and inadequate. All of my wounds came up, the old feelings of not being good enough, of self-judgment. I was in a sea of despair. And so I said a prayer:

"Dear Mother Father God, Goddess,

I need help – big time. I feel that I'm drowning in a sea of despair. Only feelings of judgment, not being good enough, are filling my mind and space. I'm having to breathe deeply. I can't see my way out. I feel that I am an energy drain, taking, not giving to the space. That I have wasted opportunities to shine and to grow. I feel disappointed with myself. I feel back at square one."

Minutes after I wrote this message to Spirit, I received a text from a friend, asking how I was. I was expecting Archangel Michael to come down and save me but, in that moment, help was sent in the form of a text. I answered it, telling my friend the complete truth. He called me straight away and, in the middle of a busy, noisy airport, I heard the words I needed to hear. My support had come in the form of an Earth angel and I was open to receive what was gifted to me in that moment.

◎   Start with an authentic heartfelt prayer or wish and ask Spirit for help.

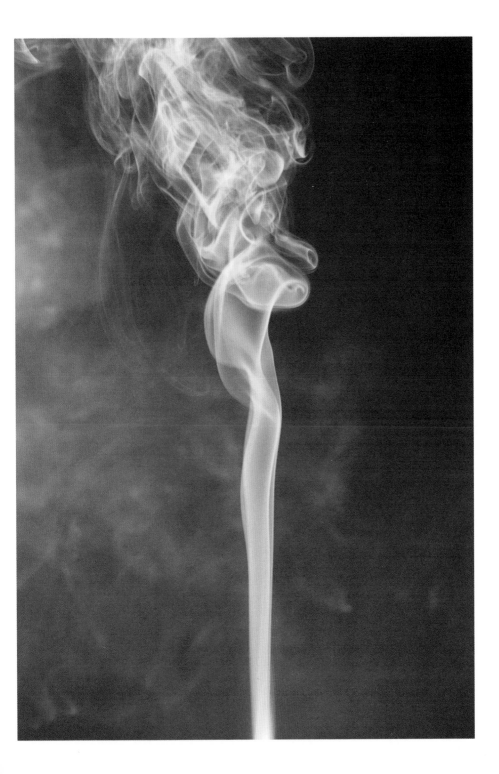

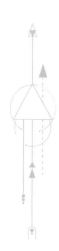

Reset Your Fight-or-Flight

Our fight-or-flight response is activated when we are in fearful or stressful situations. When our ancestors were hunter-gatherers, this response was very helpful, as it told them when to run from a situation and when to stay and fight. But because of all the modern-day western civilization stresses, many people have this mechanism activated 24/7. This means that the body is constantly producing adrenaline and cortisol, hormones that make you feel hyper-aware of any danger that might be around. You jump at the smallest thing. You sleep, but do not rest deeply. Your mind runs wild. Meditation and stillness are very difficult. Your world no longer feels safe.

Here is a process that can be used to reset your flight-or-flight response; it was shared with me via a teacher at the Pampamesayok Shaman School, which teaches ancient wisdom for empowered modern living.

Ingredients

a comfortable space, with pillows and blankets to create a warm and safe environment

- Open sacred space (see page 32).

- Lie down and get warm and cosy, with pillows under your head and knees if that's comfortable for you. Wrap yourself in a warm blanket or just get into bed.

- Take a couple of deep, cleansing breaths and begin by placing your left hand on your heart space. Continue taking long, deep breaths, then say out loud in your softest, most soothing voice:

  "Mama loves me, Mama loves me, Mama loves me."

- You are speaking to Mama Earth. Every time you say these words, invite your body to soften and feel the rhythm of your heart attuning to the rhythm of Mama Earth. Feel sweet, Divine, Earth Mother energy pouring into your heart.

- Imagine warm, nourishing and re-energizing light coming from the Cosmos. In a soft voice speak the words,

  "Papa loves me, Papa loves me, Papa loves me."

- Feel yourself being bathed in radiant light, speaking to infinite light.

- You are calling on your Earth Mother and Sun Father, who will always be there for you, nurturing and loving you.

- Rest here as long as you need to, until you feel the deep atonement and harmonizing of your heart with that of the sacred love of the Great Mother.

- Now, with your left hand still on your heart space, place your right hand on your belly. Then repeat again:

  "Mama loves me, Mama loves me, Mama loves me."

- Every time you say these words invite your body to soften and attune to the rhythm of Mama Earth.

- Notice how your body feels and then again imagine the warm, nourishing and re-energizing light coming from the Cosmos. In a soft voice speak the words:

  "Papa loves me, Papa loves me, Papa loves me."

- Feel yourself being bathed in radiant light and feel the love of Source.

- Stay here as long as you need. This is a sacred resetting of your primal love space. You will feel a deep return to peace, love and harmony in your system.

- Rest as long as you need in the sweet loving Mother Father energy. If you doze off for a little bit, perfect. When you feel complete, offer gratitude to Mama Earth and Father Sky for their love and support.

- Close sacred space (see page 32).

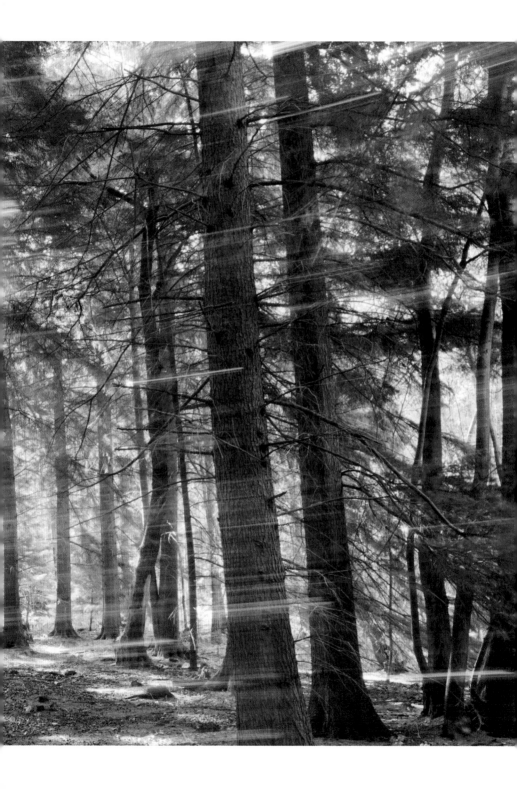

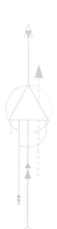

Sand Painting

When I studied the medicine wheel at the Four Winds Society, I was taught a process called sand painting that involves working with the Earth and pieces of Nature. A sand painting is a powerful tool to assist with healing, to give form to the inner pieces we are working on, giving a visual representation of change.

Often when we are in an emotional process it can be all-consuming. This practice is brilliant for getting out of the mind and into the mythic.

I was recently on a course and many deep-rooted layers were coming to the surface – it was very painful and emotional. I knew that the only thing I could do was take my process to the Earth and work with what was coming up on a mythic level.

The layers that were coming up were all around my unhealed feminine – again, it was deep-rooted feelings of not being good enough, doubting my self-worth, doubting my ability, really giving myself a hard time; then the following day there were layers of unhealed masculine all around, making me feel unsafe and not trusting. I was consumed by these feelings and I could not come back to my centre.

At the end of the day, I walked to a nearby ancient wood, and as I walked I set my intention to create a sand painting. I looked down at the path and found a phallic-shaped stick. I thought, "Oh, wow, this is perfect to honour my inner masculine." As I continued, I found feathers, leaves and sticks that I gathered. Then deep in the woods I saw a tree with an opening at the base that reminded me of the womb: the top of the opening was even shaped like a yoni. I knew this was the perfect spot to create my sand painting and bring healing to my inner feminine and inner masculine.

To begin with, I just sat by the tree, allowing my breath to slow down, my body to settle and open into presence.

Once I felt connected, I opened sacred space, calling on all the elements and my Spirit teams. I called on Mama Earth to support me, Father Sun with his alchemical fire of transformation; I called on the sacred waters of the land for their cleansing and purification; I called on the element of air, honouring every breath, and the element of ether, the energy that connects us all together. I asked the elemental beings and the Spirits of the land, my personal Spirit teams and lineages, to be present and I called on archangels and angels to surround me with their light, love and grace.

I found a selection of curved sticks to make an enclosed area around the opening at the base of the tree; then inside this enclosed space I began to make offerings. I took each item piece by piece and blew in my prayers. I took the phallic-shaped stick and blew in prayers for healing my inner masculine – may it be brought into balance and harmony. The feather representing my inner feminine – may she be brought into balance and harmony. And so on. Once all my prayers were in the painting, I felt a sense of release and relief that something inside me had shifted.

I was no longer crazy with emotions. I felt calm. As my course was a week long, I knew I wanted to work with this process over the week, so I kept my sacred space open. As I walked back through the woods I came to an open field where I saw two deer, a stag and a doe. I knew this was a symbolic message representing the masculine and feminine: deer are symbols of gentleness and kindness and are here to walk the path of love. That was the perfect message for me in that moment.

As the week went on, I continued to take issues to my sand painting, every time finding an item from Nature to represent that which was coming up for healing. Each time I would place these in the painting, allowing the Earth to work her magic.

On the last day I found that a spider had spun her web over the entrance to the opening of the tree. It looked as though the web was a guardian, holding in place all the pieces I had asked for healing, confirming that the work was done. It was a beautiful moment that made my heart sing. The spider is one of the representations of the Divine feminine and I felt she was weaving a connection between the mundane and the mythic worlds.

When we work in this way we are taking our healing out of ordinary everyday life and into another dimension, where healing can occur.

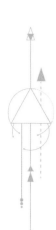

Creating a Sand Painting

Ingredients

a place in Nature, objects that you have gathered in Nature (feathers, sticks, pine cones – anything you come across that appeals to you), an issue or issues that you would like to take into the mythic realm

◎ Set your intention to find a suitable place in Nature.

◎ Mark out the area for your sand painting with sticks. You might like to create a circle at the base of the tree.

◎ Sit in your spot and invite your body to soften. Taking long, deep breaths and closing your eyes, bring yourself into presence.

◎ Open sacred space (see page 32).

◎ Consider which of your items from Nature represent the different parts of yourself that you are working through. Then, taking one object at a time, blow your prayers and wishes into it and place it within the circle. Allow yourself to be guided intuitively on where to place each item. Keep going until you feel complete.

◎ Leave the sacred space over your sand painting open and return to it every day, either to add a new item, if something has come up, or to see if you feel guided to move anything within the circle. See if natural elements such as the wind or rain have moved anything. See if anything has grown or if any animals have added a feature (like my spider's web).

◎ Take time to digest what has shifted and materialized. What do you read from the changes that have occurred naturally?

◎ Check in with yourself. How do you feel about the part of yourself you took to the sand painting?

◎ When you have finished working with the sand painting, close sacred space (see page 32) and return all the items back to Nature.

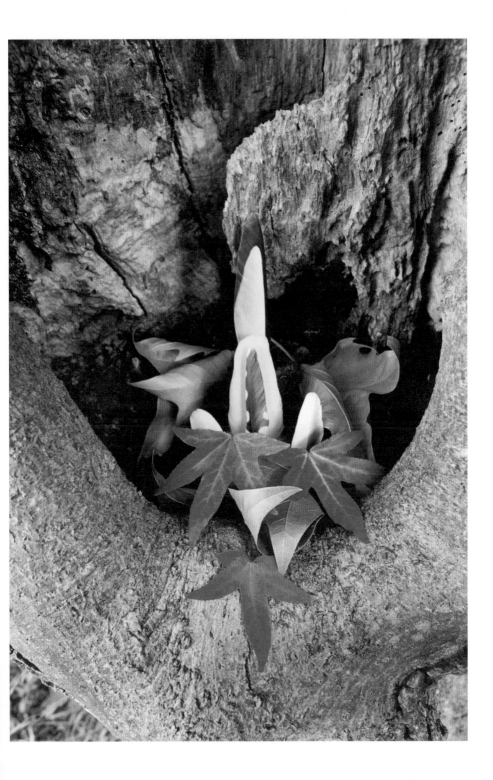

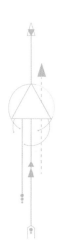

Calling on Your Angels

I was walking with a friend once and she said, "I don't believe in angels." At the top of my voice I shouted uncontrollably, "WHAT?!" Not because I was annoyed – I was just so shocked, because I am such a strong believer. You might have heard or even said, "I'll believe it when I see it." But what about "Believe it and you'll see it", as another friend once said to me?

What are angels? I believe angels are light beings that are based in a dimension living at a higher frequency than us. I believe there are many light beings that are just waiting to help and support us, and all we need to do is ask. Whenever I feel afraid or in need of extra support, I call on my angels.

◎ You can call on your angels by saying something like this:

"Dear Angels, I welcome you into my life, thank you for surrounding me with your light, love and grace, thank you for guiding and supporting me. Thank you for helping me with .... "

◎ Notice how you feel when you have said these words. What do you notice in your body, in your thoughts? How do your emotions feel? Recognize the sense of when your angels are with you.

Quick Connect and Let It All Go

This is a super-fast, plug-in meditation to connect to the Earth, to let go of what you need to, and to refill with Earth energy.

◎   Close your eyes and take a couple of breaths. Set your intention to connect with the crystalline core of the Earth.

◎ Send a ground cord from the base of your spine, wrapping it around the core of the Earth; feel a grounding tug as if Mama Earth is holding on to you.

◎ Choose to let go of the energy of the situation that you are carrying. Feel this energy drain from your body, feel the sensation of being emptied.

◎ Then invite Earth energy to come up from her crystalline core, all the way up your cord. Feel exquisite golden liquid light entering into your body, filling you from the tips of your toes to the top of your head.

◎ Offer gratitude to Mama Earth for her service, love and support.

Shake Shift Your Mood

You know some mornings you wake up feeling grumpy for no particular reason? On those days, movement can be your medicine. Some days it's yoga, some days it's dancing and some days it's shaking.

Shaking is one of my absolute favourites; you can't ever do it wrong! There is nothing to achieve, no move to aspire to. It's just shaking around to music you love. When we shake, we are releasing physical stress and tension, moving energy through our bodies, shaking off feelings and emotions ready to be released, which brings inner stillness.

Some mornings I just want to do a quick shake, so I put some music on and let my body move, relaxing into the movements, shaking every part of me. When I feel complete, I sit in silence, allowing my body to absorb the energy I have created.

Ingredients

music

◎ Shake your body, every single part of you! When you feel buzzing and humming around you, this is chi, your life-force energy. Enjoy it! Notice your emotions; see if anything has shifted for you.

◎ Then sit in stillness.

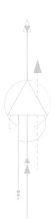

Overwhelmed

Oh goodness, we all know what it's like when everything gets on top of us and we can't see the wood for the trees. It's all just too much – where to begin, what to do?

When I feel completely overwhelmed and riddled with anxiety, I close everything down, shut my laptop, turn off my phone, shut the door, close my eyes. I bring myself back to my breath and focus on my belly. It's nothing fancy, I just slow myself right down, bring myself back inside and it works a treat!

◎ Close your laptop, put down your phone. Find a space just for yourself.

◎ Close your eyes. Slow down your breath and bring your breath into your belly.

◎ Take long, slow breaths. Breathe in for seven counts and out for seven counts. Slow down.

◎ Stay here until you feel yourself again, then come back to your centre.

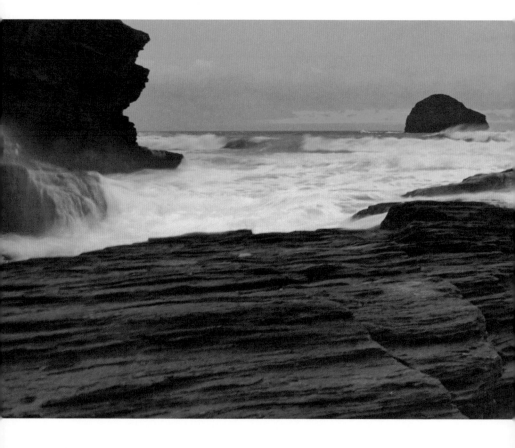

Levity Is the Best Medicine

It's easy to take ourselves way too seriously. As I said earlier, when I started on my spiritual path I became very strict and serious about everything. My papa actually said to me one day, "Chloe, be careful you don't turn into a bore." You can only imagine how livid that made me, especially when I was so busy being serious!

Levity really is one of the best medicines. Nowadays I notice that I laugh a lot and most of the time I'm laughing about how ridiculous I am. I find myself very entertaining. Laughing and playing are powerful keys.

- Play, be silly, find things that make you laugh, dance, jump around. I find spending time in Nature brings out the playfulness in me.

- Make up a song, create a dance, spend time with people you know you can laugh with!

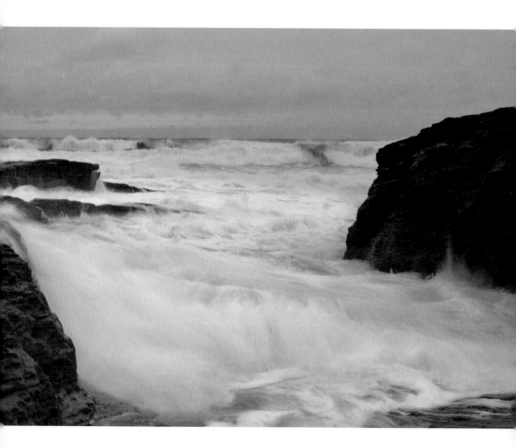

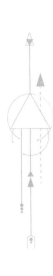

Choosing Your Medicine

I was stung by a wasp on the sole of my right foot and a couple of days later it was still inflamed, hot, red and itchy. I knew I shouldn't scratch, but I just couldn't help myself – those couple of seconds when I scratched were bliss. But as soon as I stopped, the itching, swelling and hotness came back with even more force and were even more irritating.

Then I decided to put my foot under cold water. Ahh, this soothed it, but only for a short while – I had to keep going back. In between I wanted to scratch again, but I thought, "No, don't go for the quick fix, go back to the one that supports, soothes and nourishes."

While this was happening I was having an "aha" moment. I had been feeling sad and upset that my relationship had ended, and all I wanted to do was text and be in touch with my past partner. But then I thought: it's just like scratching the itch – it will be blissful for one minute and then afterward I will be even more sore! Don't do it. Go back to the place that soothes and nourishes. Go back to Spirit – this is the relationship that will always be there for you. Nourish that relationship, feed that relationship, give time and priority to that relationship. Go as many times as you like: the Source is limitless. Profound – all for a wasp sting!

The Story of the Murky Pond

One day I woke up in a terribly grumpy mood. So I took myself for a walk to the woods. I usually take the path to the right, but this day I decided that I wasn't going to – I chose to walk to the left. I didn't really know where I was going, and as I walked I came across a bridge. I was still grumbling and I talked out loud to the trees, telling them what I was so cross about. Then all of a sudden, I came across a very small pond full of really murky, grey, dirty-looking water. I looked at the pond and thought, "You are a very dirty pond", but I stayed looking at it for a while and all of a sudden my perspective shifted. On the surface of the water all I could see were the reflections of the trees, all the different shapes of the leaves and the light cascading down. This murky pond became captivating. I couldn't take my eyes off it – the pond had become radiantly beautiful. I could no longer see the pond as dirty; I could only see a temple of light and trees and shapes. It was beyond beautiful. It was the exact message I needed to receive in that moment, to help me shift my perspective about the issue that was bothering me.

Are you looking at the dirty pond water? Or are you looking at the radiant beauty that is reflected? What are you looking at?

Nature's Temple

I mentioned this before in Staying Connected (see page 150), as I believe the most nourishing, self-caring thing we can do for ourselves is to spend time in Nature. Whether it is walking by the sea, walking through a forest or woods, climbing over rocks or strolling through the park, Nature has the unique ability to bring us back into our centre. Any time I feel out of sorts, the best place for me is with the trees. If I have a problem, I'll walk and talk to the trees. I'll often lie down under a tree. I always receive fresh new perspectives and feel a whole lot better than when I started.

◎ Take yourself for a walk in Nature. Choose to connect to the Nature around you.

◎ Do you receive any messages from looking at the trees, the flowers, the sea? How do you feel?

◎ If you have a problem, speak it out loud to the trees, ask for their advice. See what messages come to you.

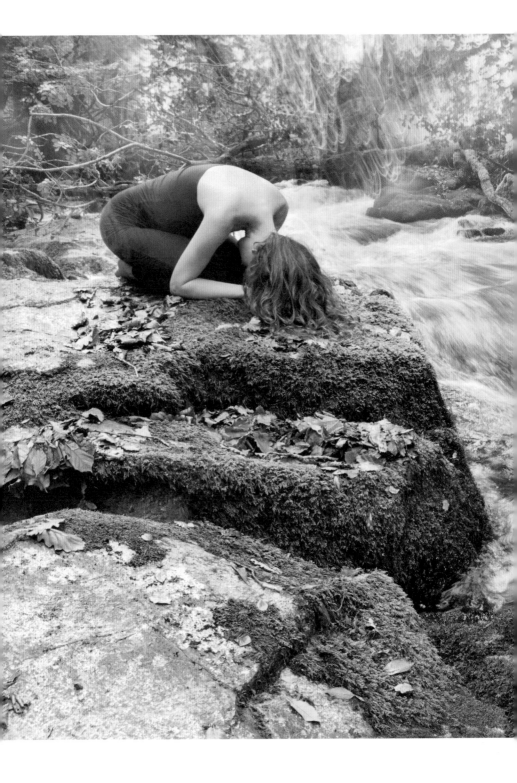

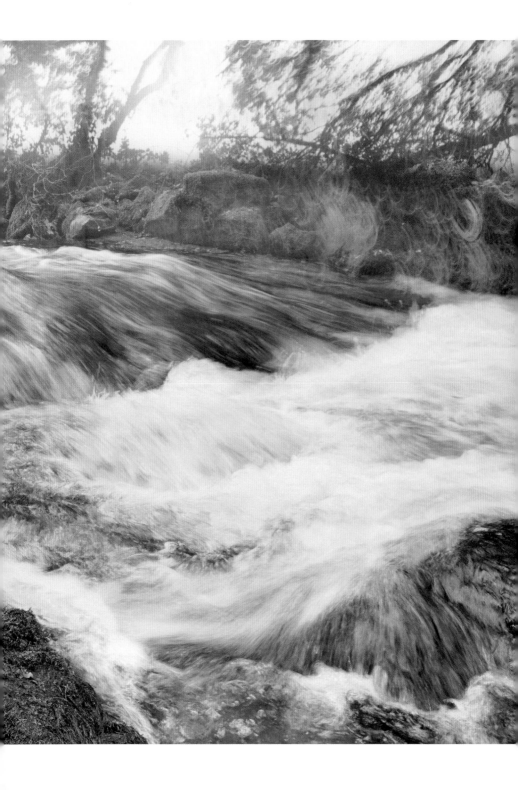

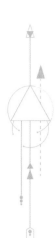

Resources

Palo Santo is a fragrant wood that grows in South America, and is known as "Holy Wood". When the wood is burned, the smoke is believed to have healing and spiritual properties, and to be a powerful energetic cleanser.

Usage: Light one stick of palo santo. The flame will go out and the stick will smoke, but you may need to light the stick a couple more times as it does not smoke for long. Use as much as is required for your ritual or ceremony.

White sage is an evergreen shrub that predominantly grows in high altitude desert ecosystems across the United States (particularly California). It is believed to be a sacred plant ally for cleansing, purifying, protection and for creating sacred space.

Usage: Light the bundle of sage, then blow out the flame so that the sage smokes. Hold a fireproof bowl underneath to catch the ash and do your blessing and clearing/cleansing while the sage smokes. Once finished, press the sage into the bowl to stop the smoking.

Note: While palo santo and white sage are incredible healing tools, they are also over-harvested. It is important to always buy from sustainable and ethical resources.

Water from a sacred site: water is in itself sacred, but there are particular sites around the world that are known as holy because of their abilities to bring healing and nourishment to the mind, body and soul. These include the Chalice Well and the White Spring in Glastonbury and St Nectans Glen waterfall in Tintagel (all in south-west England), the spring from the grotto in Lourdes (France), Lake Atitlán (Guatemala), Crater Lake (Oregon, United States), the River Ganges (India), the sacred waterfall in Abadiania at John of God (Brazil). Water from a place in Nature – rivers, lakes, waterfalls, springs and wells – is also sacred.

MyMoon Power Essential Oils are pure essential anointing oils for menstrual empowerment. The oils assist women in expanding their awareness of their own inner power, beauty, radiance and magic, while honouring the sacredness of the phases of the monthly cycle: www.mymoonpower.com

Moon Cups are reusable, medical-grade silicon cups that are inserted into the vagina to collect the blood during menstruation. They are an eco-friendly alternative to tampons and sanitary pads.

Edible Essential Oils are food-grade essential oils that you can ingest.

Ceremonial Grade Cacao is formed when cacao – grown with the intention of being used for ceremony – has been through minimal processing and none of the butter is stripped away. The beans are lightly toasted or sundried and then made into a paste once the husks are removed by hand.

www.thefourwinds.com
Combining ancient Shamanic wisdom teachings with nutrition, biology and neuroscience, the Light Body School programme at the Four Winds Society offers Shamanic healing and energy medicine.

www.redschool.net
Alexandra Pope and Sjanie Hugo Wurlitzer are the co-founders of Red School, a women's leadership, creativity and spiritual approach based on the feminine way of the menstrual cycle.

www.purerevitalizingenergy.com
Stephen Feely teaches ancient wisdom for empowered modern living at the Pampamesayok Shaman School. Chloe Isidora is also on the faculty.

www.oo.academy
The O&O Academy is a philosophy and meditation school for the transformation of human consciousness.

www.crystallinegoddess.earth
www.blissrox.com
Aravel Garduno is a powerful healer and gifted conscious medium specializing in Crystalline Consciousness Matrix. She also creates exquisite fine jewellery.

www.devaproject.com
Jami Deva is a Shaman, guide and mentor deeply influenced by the Sufi path of love and devotion, Qigong and mystical arts.

www.soundawakening.co.uk
Louise Shiels from Sound Awakening is a sacred Cacao Gong ceremonialist, sound healer and reiki master.

www.yvonnefuchs.com
Yvonne Fuchs is a mentor and creative business coach, and co-founder of the Zen of Business.

www.emmacannon.co.uk
Emma Cannon is a fertility and women's health expert, acupuncturist and author.

www.theriteofthewomb.com
The Rite of the Womb: the 13th Rite of the Munay-Ki, a lineage of womb blessing.

www.secretyogaclub.co.uk
The Secret Yoga Club offers yoga, workshops and retreats that encourage creativity and being your unique self.

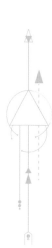

Further Reading

Cannon, E. (2017) *Fertile: Nourish and Balance Your Body Ready for Baby Making*, London: Vermilion

Dinsmore-Tuli, U. (2014) *Yoni Shakti: A Woman's Guide to Power and Freedom Through Yoga and Tantra*, London: YogaWords

Hugo Wurlitzer, S. and Pope, A. (2017) *Wild Power: Discover the Magic of Your Menstrual Cycle and Awaken the Feminine Path of Power*, London: Hay House

Kent, T. L. (2011) *Wild Feminine: Finding Power, Spirit & Joy in the Female Body*, London: Atria Books/Beyond Words

Villoldo, A. (2018) *The Heart of the Shaman: Stories and Practices of the Luminous Warrior*, London: Hay House

Villoldo, A. (2015) *One Spirit Medicine: Ancient Ways to Ultimate Wellness*, London: Hay House

Winston, S. (2010) *Women's Anatomy of Arousal: Secret Maps to Buried Pleasure*, Emeryville CA: Mango Garden Press

Index

(page numbers in *italic* refer to photographs and diagrams)

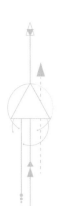

Acknowledgments

Thank you to my ever-loving and supportive family: Nicky Kerman, Juanita Kerman, Sasha Kerman, Gaywood and Casa K.

Thank you Gustavo Papaleo for all your passionate creativity, beautiful photographs and for working above and beyond.

Thank you Richard Howard, Yvonne Fuchs and Emma Cannon for your endless support and encouragement.

Thank you to my muse for the abundance of content creation.

Thank you St Nectans Glen for allowing us to take photographs on your sacred land.

Thank you to all my beloved soul sisters for all your love, support, tears and laughter.

Thank you to Valeria Huerta and Olivia Percival for making this all happen.

Extra special thank you to Kate Adams and Ella Parsons for all your support, guidance and patience!

Thank you to all my teachers and guides, to name a few: Aravel Garduno, Alberto Villoldo, Marcela Lobos, Jami Deva, Wendy, Stephen Feely, Lokpal, Alexandra Pope and Sjanie Hugo Wurlitzer.

And biggest thank you of all to my Spirit teams and lineages.

About the Author

After 10 years working as a fashion editor, Chloe Isidora followed her heart into the world of healing, mysticism and magic. Now trained in Shamanism, Crystalline Consciousness and Divine Feminine Empowerment, Chloe centres her work around transformation, empowerment and self-love. She works one-to-one and hosts regular events. Chloe's self-care and self-love practices can be easily integrated into daily life, to bring a deeper awareness of one's inner wisdom and intuition. Nourishing a sense of connection with the natural world, these practices will encourage readers to live from a place of truth.

www.chloeisidora.com